The First Case of Lupus

❖

SYLVIA MCALLISTER

Copyright © 2021 Sylvia McAllister
All rights reserved
First Edition

NEWMAN SPRINGS PUBLISHING
320 Broad Street
Red Bank, NJ 07701

First originally published by Newman Springs Publishing 2021

ISBN 978-1-63692-918-7 (Paperback)
ISBN 978-1-63692-919-4 (Digital)

Printed in the United States of America

Introduction

The victim of this deadly disease is a twenty-two-year-old Black female. She has three children and is living on welfare. When she first got sick, the doctors didn't know what was wrong with her. The disease, lupus, took control of her body, and they had no idea what it was or what to do about it.

We lived in Riverdale, a community in Dillon, South Carolina, in a big yellow stone house with our mother, Thelma, and our aunt Kitty. There were six of us kids. Sterling, the youngest, was thirteen. I was fifteen. Debra was eighteen and married when she was sixteen. Randy was twenty. Gent was twenty-two, and Na was twenty-five.

It was December 31, 1977. It was also New Year's Eve. There were only three of us at home—that is, three of our mother's kids. Gent's three kids lived with us too. Tula was five. Von was four, and Ricky was two and a half.

Debra and her husband, Andrew, lived across town. Gent wasn't married, but she did have a place of her own. She lived down the road from us on the corner. Charlie Taylor, her boyfriend, stayed with her. She had been going with him for seven months.

Na was married to Dora Page. They had two kids, Junior and Tina. Things didn't work out between them, and he moved back home.

Mama, Sterling, and I were on welfare and food stamps. Gent had her and the kids on it too. When Na moved back home, Mama didn't report it because he said he wouldn't be there very long. She told him not to worry about it. Getting on welfare was easy then. You didn't have to go through all kinds of changes like you do now.

Na and Randy had good jobs. They both worked at Buck Creek Industries. Na was a fixer in maintenance, and Randy was a machine operator. Later that year, in 1978, both of them got job promotions. Na became a supervisor, and Randy became a fixer.

Gent had to go to the hospital early on New Year's Eve morning before daylight. She was crying. She had Charlie come to the house and get Mama. Everybody was asleep, but Mama got up on the second knock.

When she opened the door, Charlie said, "Gent said come there. She hurtin'."

"She hurtin'? Hurtin' where?"

"She didn't say. She just told me to come and get you."

"Let me get ma coat. I'm comin'."

Mama got her coat and went back with him. Gent was still in bed, crying. Mama asked her where was she hurting, and she said that she was just hurting. Mama told Charlie to help her get ready and that she was going to wake up Na and get him to take them to the hospital. Na got ready and, on the way out, picked them up.

When they got to the hospital, they took her in, examined her, and later put her in a room. Aunt Kitty had gone up there earlier that morning to spend the day with her. I got my boyfriend, Bobby, to take me to the hospital to see her.

When we walked in, I said, "Hey, girl. Have ya stopped hurtin' yet?"

She said, "Just a little bit. I ain't hurtin' like I was this mornin' and last night, not since they put me on this kidney machine."

"Well, you know that old sayin', 'Whatever you be doin' when the New Year come in, you'll be doin' it all year long.' That mean you'll be in here all of '78."

"Girl, don't talk like that. I ain't never planned on comin' here." Then she looked over at Bobby and said, "Hey there, Rabbit."

He said, "Hey, Gent, how you doin'?"

"I'll make it, I reckon."

"With the help of the Lord, you'll make it."

"Yep, I feel pretty good now."

Then Aunt Kitty asked me, "Where ya mama?"

I said, "She went up town to buy Gent a gown. She said that she couldn't find one at her house."

"I got some gowns. She just ain't look in the right place. But I could always use a new one."

Aunt Kitty said, "Is she comin' up here?"

THE FIRST CASE OF LUPUS

"She said she was as soon as she got the stuff she had to get for Gent," I said.

"Oh, I'll go home with y'all then."

"Okay."

We stayed a few more minutes and left. We met Mama at a store on our way home. She was on her way to see Gent. She told me to tell Na to go pick her up at eighty thirty because she was getting dropped off. When she got there, Gent told her that the doctor had been in.

Mama asked her, "What did he say?"

"Nothin', but I can go home tomorrow."

"I'm glad to hear that. Ain't you?"

"Shine yeah, you know I am."

"I guess that mean ya kidneys doin' pretty good by theyself."

"He said that it won't as bad as it coulda been."

"Is he gon' give ya some medicine just in case it start up again?"

"I hope so."

The next day, Gent came home from the hospital, and we went back to school. Mama asked her if she was coming home with her. Gent said no because she was feeling good. Mama told her if she started feeling bad again, to let her know. She also told her to take her medicine.

She took her medicine, but there were still some problems. It was the middle of January, and it was pouring down rain. It was up in the middle of the day. I didn't go to school that day because of the rain. Gent hadn't been over, so I went to her house to see why. When I got there, she was in the bed balled up in a knot under the covers.

I said, "God, it's cold in here. What happen to ya fire?"

She heated with wood just like we did.

"Why, is it gone out?"

"Yeah. I'll put some more wood in it."

"There ain't no mo'. Charlie got to get some."

"Is that why y'all in the bed?"

"That's part of it. Ma head's hurtin', and ma knees achin'."

"Ya knees?"

"Yeah."

"Why don't cha go to the house?"

"Nah, I'ma stay here and lie down for a while."

"I'll get some wood from the house if you want me to."

"Yeah, bring me a few pieces."

I went home but not to get wood. I told Mama about her instead. When I walked in the door, Mama asked me what Gent was doing.

"Nothin'," I said. "She over there in the bed."

"In the bed! What she doin' in the bed?"

"She said she was hurtin', and she ain't got no wood either."

"None? I swear. Where Charlie? In the bed too?"

"Nope. I told her to come over here, but she said that she was gonna stay in the bed."

"Go back over there and tell that girl to come here. Her ass a freeze over there wit no fire. Tell Charlie to come wit her."

"She might not come 'cause you talk junk about her gettin' yo' wood last week."

"Just go tell her what I said."

"I'll go back in a minute. Let me warm up first."

I stood by the heater for a while and then got my coat and went back to her house. When I walked in the door, she was coming out of the kitchen walking slowly.

I said, "Mama said for y'all to come to the house."

"What she send for us for? She talk shit about us last week."

"I told her that."

"What she say then?"

"Go'n and tell that girl I said come here. She'll freeze over there with no fire in that house."

"Getcha coat, Charlie."

I said, "I know you was goin'."

"Yeah. Maybe she got somethin' that I can take for this pain."

"I believe we got some alcohol and Anacin."

"I don't care what it is as long as it helps me." They put on their coats and toboggans. Then we went back to the house in the rain.

When we walked in the door, Gent went straight to the heater to get warm. Mama looked at her and laughed.

She said, "I shoulda letcha stay over there in that cold house."

THE FIRST CASE OF LUPUS

Gent had a little smile on her face as she said, "What you send for me for then? I coulda stayed."

"Child, go'n. A little bit longer, you'da come over here on ya own."

"I sho woulda."

"When ya knees and ya head started botherin' ya?"

"This mornin'."

"It might be arthritis," said Mama.

"That might be what it is."

"Take some Anacin and lie on this chair. Maybe it'll ease off."

"All right."

Mama got her a quilt and put it on the sofa for her. Gent stood by the heater a little while longer and then got on the sofa and lay down. We watched soap operas the rest of the day.

Days passed, and each day was just like the other.

If Gent didn't have a headache, she was complaining about her joints aching. Every now and then, she looked swollen.

We had to look at her closely to tell if she was. To me, she seemed to be losing a little weight. It seemed like I was the only one to notice it. Nobody else in the family ever said anything about it. For some reason, they used to say I was big for my age. I didn't think so, but Gent and I wore the same size in clothes and shoes. On my birthday, when she borrowed a pair of my pants to wear to the club, I noticed that they were baggy on her. We went out together for a little while and had a good time. We came back home before eleven. Gent said that she wasn't feeling very good, so Bobby and I took her home.

"Why don't cha go to the doctor and let him check and see if he know why yo' legs achin' like that," I said on the way home.

She said, "It don't really bother me that bad. After I get off ma feet for a while, they ease off."

"If it was me, I'd sho go and have one to look at me."

"Me too," said Bobby.

"I hate to spoil ya night, sis, but I just can't hang no longer."

"That's all right. Me and Bobby gon' go back out for a little while longer."

"I enjoyed maself while I was out there though. I woulda had more fun if that wor'some-ass Joe Ward woulda stayed out my face."

I said, "Why don't cha tell Charlie?"

Bobby laughed.

She said, "You know better than that. I hate to see Charlie get on old Joe. He was high when I left. He might be 'sleep."

When we got to the house, she got out of the car.

Before I closed the car door, I said, "You still ought to go to the doctor and have yo'self examined."

Bobby said, "Yeah. You never know what he might find. It's best to know than not to know."

"That's right 'cause, if they find out what it is, they can catch it before it get out of hand," I said.

"I told y'all not to worry. I'll be all right."

I figured that she knew what she was talking about. So we let her go on in, and we left. When I got back home that night, Mama was still up.

"Gent come home wit you?" she asked.

"We brought her home at eleven. She said that she was hurtin' in her legs again."

"Why she didn't come over here, ya reckon?"

"I don't know. Charlie was up waitin' on her when she got home."

"Well, I'll go check on her tomorrow. Long as he there wit her, I ain't worried about her. He'll let me know if she ain't feelin' good."

"Well, I'ma sit out here in the yard wit Bobby Gene for a while. I'll be back in in a few minutes."

"That's you. I'm goin' back to bed."

"Don't lock the door 'cause I ain't gon' be nowhere but in the yard."

She said okay and went to bed. The next morning, Mama got up still talking about Gent.

By the time I walked through the curtain to my room, she said, "How long did Gent say her legs had been hurtin'?"

"She didn't. Last night, she said that she was ready to go because they was hurtin'."

"Well, I'ma go see 'bout her."

When Mama got there, Gent got up to open the door. Charlie was still in bed.

Gent said, "What in the world you doin' stirrin' early this mornin'?"

"I come to see how you doin'."

"I'm doin' fine. What's supposed to be wrong wit me?"

"Silver Jean told me that yo' legs was botherin' ya last night."

"They was, but I feel fine now."

"Well, I'ma go then. If you need anything, let me know."

"Okay."

Later in the day, she came over to the house. We talked for a long time.

"Girl, my head hurt me so bad sometime I feel like I'm goin' crazy," she said.

"If it's hurtin' that bad, you won't be able to work in tobacco this time, will ya?"

"I can as long as it ain't too bad."

"I don't know. You know that sun ain't gon' do nothin' but make it worse 'cause there ain't no shade on that tractor."

"I'ma just try it for a while, and if I can't do it, me and you'll have to change places."

That sounded good to me. Anything was better than pickin' up leaves.

On the first of February, Gent got her check. She went uptown and bought herself a pair of pants and a blouse.

She asked me to go with her, and she said that she'd buy me something too. I saw a pretty beige wool skirt. I told her that I wanted it instead of pants. She decided to get herself one too. I picked up a size 10 and went in the dressing room to try it on. It was a perfect fit. Gent tried one in the same size, and it was too big. She put it back and got a size 8. It was just right. I was surprised but not as much as she was.

I looked at her and said, "See, you did lose weight."

"Ah, hush," she said.

She paid for the clothes, and we left. On the way home, I asked her if she was on a diet.

She said no but that she didn't eat as much as she used to.

I didn't really pay any attention to what she was saying. I was busy trying to decide when I was going to wear my new skirt.

Gent wasn't sick every day. Most of the time, she was like the old Gent we all know, who was always talking trash to everybody. She kept something going.

On Valentine's Day, Charlie got her some candy. As soon as she got it, she brought it over to the house and gave most of it to the kids. Mama ate a couple of pieces.

When I asked her if I could have some, she said, "No. You better wait till Bobby Gene bring yours."

I sat at home all day, waiting for him to bring it.

When he did get there, he didn't have any candy. I went to Gent's house and got some of hers. She teased me because I didn't get any. I told her that he was taking me out to dinner instead.

"Where y'all goin', or is it any of my business?" she said.

I said, "To Hardee's or Wiener King."

"Bring me a burger back, and I'll give you some mo' candy when ya get back."

I said okay and left.

We didn't stay gone too long. When we got back, we went to Gent's house to give her the sandwich she wanted.

I got her a big deluxe. I stayed to see if she was going to eat it. She did, just as if she had been eating all the time.

I looked at her and said, "I thought you said that you didn't eat as much as you used to."

"I don't, but that was good. Sometimes I can go days without eatin' anything. It's like ma appetite comes and goes."

"I like the size that you are now, just as long as you don't get any skinnier."

"I'ma try not to. If I can help it, I ain't."

I went into the kitchen to get myself some Kool-Aid. I looked in the cabinet to see what she had to snack on.

THE FIRST CASE OF LUPUS

I said, "This food you got last month sho is lastin' a long time. It would be all right if it could last this long at home."

She and Bobby laughed.

"It'll soon be time for you to go grocery again. Charlie must not be eatin' either."

"Yeah. He eatin'. Next month, I won't have that much to get."

Bobby said, "I know you glad about that, ain't cha?"

"You know that's right."

"You got a birthday next month. Whatcha gon' do, have a party?" I asked.

"Nah. I'll probably go out and party a little bit. You gon' go wit me?"

"Yeah. I reckon that depends on what I have planned. Ain't that right, Bob?"

"I don't know. That's you talkin'."

"Well, Rabbit can party wit us too. You know that. The more the merrier. I'ma sell some of my stamps so I can have some money that night."

"Well, I know that I ain't gonna have none," I said.

"Like I said, don't worry 'bout it."

Gent's birthday was March 26.

All that month, Mama walked around the house, saying, "That gal of mine gon' want that chocolate cake for her birthday, so I might as well get ma stuff I'ma need."

Three days before her birthday, she came over to the house. She never did mention anything to Mama about a cake, and that was strange. This was the first time she had not asked for a cake. She sat there for a while talking to Mama, then she got up to leave.

Mama said, "You must don't want no cake for ya birthday?"

"Why come I don't?" Gent asked.

"Well, you didn't say anything about it."

"I didn't think I had to. You know I want one."

"I figured you did. That's why I went on and got the stuff. Is you gon' pay me for it?" Mama asked, laughing.

"Yeah, pay you no 'tention."

"I knew that before I asked ya."

"Well, whatcha ask me for then?"

Mama said, "Child, go on."

Gent said, "I am," and walked out the door.

Before she reached her house, I ran up behind her and walked home with her.

I asked her, "Whatcha gettin' ready to do, cook?"

"No. I'm goin' home to lie down."

"Lie down! This time of the day?" I asked.

"Yeah, I got a headache. It ain't that bad though. I'll be back in a little while."

"Well, I'll be back later. I'm goin' to Ludy house."

"Okay."

I left, and she went on in the house to lie down. I didn't stay at Ludy's house very long before I was back, but while I was there, she and I walked up to Chucky's house so I could borrow his camera. When we got back, we went to Gent's house. Ludy was three years older than I was. We were both still like tomboys, and I know that we must have really got on Gent's nerves about taking pictures. She told us two or three times that she didn't feel up to it, but we kept at her until she said okay.

We almost took the whole pack of film. Gent acted like she still wasn't feeling very well, but she laughed along with us anyway.

When we finished, there were only two pictures left.

I told Ludy that I'd save them for tomorrow. We got the pictures and went in the house to see how they turned out. All of them came out good except one with me and Gent.

Ludy picked at me and said that I had broken the camera because it was only messed up on my side.

Mama finished the cake and had me take it over to Gent.

"Lord, that cake look good. I'll probably eat me a piece after a while," Gent said.

Ludy said, "You ain't gon' cut it till after a while?"

She said, "Why? You want some now?"

"Yeah. I 'clare that cake look good."

"Go head and cut cha a piece."

I got up and headed for the kitchen.

"I want some too," Charlie said, who was right behind us.

Gent said, "I figured you did. I'm surprised you didn't ask before Ludy did."

"She didn't give me a chance."

All of us laughed.

It was getting dark, so I walked Ludy halfway home.

She asked me if I was going out tonight, but I told her no.

I wanted to stay home and see the movie. It was one of my favorite Jerry Lewis movies.

When I got to Gent's house on my way home, she called me and told me to come there a minute. I went over to see what she wanted.

She said, "You goin' out tonight wit us like I asked ya to?"

"Where y'all goin?"

"Nowhere but Eddie's."

"I might have to pass tonight. I wanna see the movie that's comin' on."

"Girl, you can see that movie some other time."

"I'll letcha know."

"See, if it was Ludy askin' you, you would have said yeah."

"No, I wouldn't have either. She asked me to go, but I told her no."

"Well, you go'n and get ready, and we can go by her house and catch her before she go."

"I'll letcha know after I talk to Bob."

"Oh hell, go'n to the house and get ready."

I laughed and said, "Okay. I'll be back. Whatcha'll tryin' to get so clean for?"

"I ain't tryin' to get clean, and whatcha mean y'all? I don't see where I'm so clean at. I ain't got on nothin' but a blouse and a pair pants. Go'n get ready and hurry back."

I went home and got dressed. We met Kelly and his girlfriend on our way out. They were planning on getting married this month. All of us got together and went out to party. Charlie said that he would be out later on. He was just in from playing basketball and had to wash.

When we got out there, Joe Ward was there. He tried all he could to get Gent to go with him. She told him to leave her alone because Charlie was comin' out later.

He got mad and told her, "When yo' nigger ain't around, you be runnin' me down. I don't care if he is comin'. You goin' wit me tonight."

She ignored him and wasn't paying him any attention. The more she ignored him, the louder he got. When Charlie walked in, he went up to him and told him that Gent was tryin' to get him to go off with her before he walked in.

Kelly's girlfriend told Charlie that Joe was lying. Joe slapped her and told her to mind her damn business. At that time, Kelly went to find Maco.

Joe's brother Robert grabbed him by the hand and told him that he should be ashamed of himself. He got mad at him and told him to go to hell.

Gent took Ella, Kelly's girlfriend, outside. Charlie went out behind them, and Joe went out behind Charlie.

Robert got in his car and took off with his wheels spinning. Joe came out the door fussing, and his other brother Jay asked him what was wrong.

He said, "I'm gettin' ready to fuck me one up."

Jay said, "No, you ain't either. You gettin' ready to go sit down somewhere."

"You don't tell me what to do. I help raise you. You ain't got shit to do wit it. You gon' be doin' the sittin' down."

Gent had already told Jay about Joe slapping Ella.

Jay said, "Now you know that you ain't got no business hittin' on another man's wife. You gon' mess around and get killed."

"That's the motherfucker I want right there," Joe said and pointed at Charlie.

"Let him come on. I'm right here if he wants me," Charlie said.

His brother turned him loose and told him to go ahead and get his ass beaten. Joe didn't say anything else for a while.

Then Gent said, "Let's go, y'all."

Charlie said, "We ain't got to go."

"You gonna let him stop you from havin' a good time?" said Ella.

"We can go somewhere else and have a good time."

Then Joe said, "You better haul ass."

Charlie said, "I done had 'bout enough of his damn mouth."

Gent and Ella talked him into leaving. They told him not to pay Joe any attention because he was drunk.

Joe heard them talking, and he said, "I hear ya. I be damn if I'm drunk. I ain't no fool either."

They left and went home. When they told Aunt Essie, Kelly's mother, about it, she was ready to go back out there with her gun. But they talked her out of it, and they got ready to go back home in Lumberton. Essie said that it wasn't over with and that all she wanted to do was lay her eyes on Joe Ward. She was going to give him a piece of her mind.

Time passed, and more and more, Gent complained about headaches and aching in her joints. I saw that she wasn't getting any better, so I said something about it to Mama.

"Every time I go to Gent's house, she be takin' somethin' for pain."

"Whatcha talkin' 'bout?" she asked.

"For the last few weeks, she been havin' pains in her head and legs."

"This heat must be doin' it. She walked over the other day, and when she come up on the porch, she was poppin' sweat."

"She was like that before it started gettin' hot. She lost some weight too."

"I'ma go see how she doin'. If anybody call for me, tell 'em I'll call 'em back."

"Okay," I said.

When she got there, Charlie was on the chair watching a basketball game. Mama asked him where Gent was, and he said she was still lying down. Mama went into the room where she was.

"You still havin' problems, girl?"

"I just got a little headache, that's all. I took a couple of Goody's Powders."

"They ain't ease it off none?"

"A little bit. It'll probably stop after a while."

"You wanna go to the doctor?"

"No, ma'am."

"Yo' blood pressure might be high. Ya might need to get it checked."

"If I don't get no better, I will. Where Head at?"

"At the house. Oh well, I'ma go back and finish cookin'. If ya need anything, let me know."

"Okay. Tell Head to come here."

Oh yeah, Head is one of my nicknames.

"All right."

Mama left. When she walked in the door, she told me what Gent said, and I went over to see what she wanted.

We talked for a while, then I went in the kitchen to see what she had to eat. When I looked in the refrigerator, she still had half of her birthday cake left.

I said, "Girl, I know something's wrong wit you. You still got a half of chocolate cake left."

"I been meanin' to give it to them youngerns. It ain't that much. We ate most of it."

Charlie said, "I ate it till I lost the taste for it."

She said, "I'ma have to throw it out now. Don't tell Mama now."

"I ain't."

Two days later, I borrowed Chucky's camera again. I bought some more film. Gent, Sterling, Charlie, the kids, and I took some pictures. After we finished, everybody took a quick look at them. I got them together and took them home to put in my photo album. I stopped and looked at the one taken of Gent standing next to the house by herself.

She had lost a lot of weight, and I could tell.

She came to the house every day, and nobody ever said anything about her looking sick or losing weight. I figured that they just didn't want to believe that anything was seriously wrong with her. But the time came when none of us had a choice.

THE FIRST CASE OF LUPUS

When Charlie got home that night from visiting his family, I went over there for a while. I took the pictures with me. I had the one that I had taken of her on her birthday and the one that I had just taken of her that day.

I handed them to Charlie and told him to look at them together. "Didn't she lose a lot of weight?"

He said, "Yeah, and I mean a lot."

"And them pictures ain't but a month apart."

"Damn, what's wrong, babe?"

She said, "I ain't been eatin'. What do you expect?"

"I know that, and it's about time to find out why. Don't you think so?"

I said, "And find out what's causin' them headaches and achin' in ya leg joints."

"You better go to the doctor, especially if ya head givin' ya trouble."

"Yeah, I know ya right. I ain't been right since I went in the hospital for kidney failure," she said.

"I know it, and now ya havin' headaches."

Gent looked at me and said, "You got a date tonight?"

"Yeah, but it ain't time for him yet."

As soon as I said that, we saw a car light shine through the window.

Gent looked out the window and said, "It might not be time for him, but there he is."

Charlie laughed.

I said, "No, it ain't, girl?"

"Yes, it is too. See."

I looked out the window, and he was pulling up into our yard.

I said, "Well, let me go. I'll see y'all tomorrow."

By the first of April, Gent had gotten a little worse. Mama said that she was going to take her to the hospital or the doctor to find out what was wrong with her. Gent tried to talk her out of it, but Mama didn't listen to her.

Aunt Kitty said that, in a few days, we were going to start setting out tobacco. Gent wanted to help, but she wasn't able to. She said she was going to anyway.

The morning we got ready to go to work, Gent got up early. She was at the house before any of us were ready.

"Where you think you goin'?" Mama said.

"To help set out 'bacco."

"What Charlie say about that?"

"Whatcha mean 'what Charlie say'? What's he supposed to say?"

"He told you the other day that you wasn't settin' out no 'bacco."

"Charlie can't tell me what to do."

"You ain't got no business out there in that sun."

"Well, I ain't gon' make no money sittin' home lookin' at him."

"You'd rather go out there and almost kill yaself for a few dollars. Whatcha gon' do then?"

"Ain't nothin' I can do then. When ya dead, ya done?"

"Well, that's you."

"I'll be all right. When it get too hot, I'll take a break. It might not get too hot today. I'm hopin' it won't anyway."

"That bendin' ain't gon' help ya none either."

"I know."

"The way yo' head been hurtin', and you gon' go help set out 'bacco?"

"It might not be too bad. It didn't bother me none yesterday."

"That was yesterday."

"I'ma just try it today."

"You go head if you want to. I sho wouldn't."

"I got a couple of Goody's Powders in ma pocket just in case it do start."

When Mr. Jack pulled up in the yard, we all got in the car. Gent and I got in the back, and Aunt Kitty got in the front with him.

He said, "Hey, Gent, how you doin'?"

"Pretty good, Mr. Jack. How you?"

"Pretty good. Pretty good."

"That's good."

THE FIRST CASE OF LUPUS

He and Aunt Kitty talked all the way to work. Gent and I talked a little, but most of the time, she sat with her head leaned up against the window.

I asked her, "Yo' head hurtin'?"

She said, "No, not really. It's just achin' a little bit."

"Oh, I wish Cookie woulda come this mornin'."

Cookie was a friend of mine who stayed with us.

"I been meanin' to ask you why she didn't come."

"She was havin' cramps. It's her time of the month."

"I'm glad mine done come and gone."

"Me too," I said.

When we got to the tobacco beds, they had already started to work. Everybody looked up and spoke when we got out of the car. Gent was able to pull plants for a while. Then at ten, she told me that she had to go sit down for a while. I asked her if her head had started bothering her already, and she said yes.

When Aunt Kitty saw her going to sit down, she said, "It done started hurtin' ya again?"

"Yes, ma'am."

Mrs. Bell said, "How often do she have 'em?"

"They come and go," said Aunt Kitty.

"Is she been to the doctor for 'em, Kitty?" asked Mrs. Dora.

"No, not yet. Nank said she was gonna take her if it keep on botherin' her."

Nank was Mama's nickname.

Mrs. Bell said, "Well, you doin' the right thing by sittin' down. We don't wantcha failin' out on us out here."

"If it get any worse, you'll have to go home," said Mrs. Dora.

"Nank told her, to start with, not to come, but she came anyway."

Mrs. Bell told Gent, "If ya wanna go home now, Jack can take ya."

"All right, I think I better. Feel like it's tryin' to get worse. I'm havin' chills too."

"Ya might be comin' down wit a cold," said Mrs. Dora.

"No, she get like that. 'Bout a month and a half ago, she come to the house in the rain and said that she was achin' in the knee joints. Nank gave her some stuff to rub down wit. It eased her off a little bit."

"She lost a lot of weight too, Kitty. That girl don't look well a bit," said Mrs. Bell.

Mrs. Dora said, "She sho don't, but I hope she be all right."

"Nank, get her straightened out," said Aunt Kitty.

The next morning, Gent wanted to go back to work. Charlie told her that she wasn't going, but she didn't pay any attention to him. She put on her clothes and came over to the house.

Mama said, "You might as well go right back home and take them work clothes off 'cause you ain't goin' to try and pull not one plant this roomin'."

Gent got mad, but she didn't say anything. By the time Mama said that, Aunt Kitty was coming out of her room.

She looked at Gent and said, "Where you think you goin' this mornin', miss?"

Gent didn't even look up at her. She just said, "Nowhere now."

Aunt Kitty laughed and said, "You oughta knowed better than that."

Finally, we finished settin' out tobacco. After that, it seemed like time flew. Maybe it was because Gent got worse as each day passed. By the end of April, her appetite was gone completely. She had not really been eating anyway. But for the last two weeks or more, she wouldn't or couldn't eat anything. She had lost so much weight it looked like she was drying up.

Charlie didn't have a car of his own. So whenever he had to go somewhere, he asked Randy to take him, or he'd borrow the car. It was the first week in May, and Charlie was trying to find a job. He had been everywhere, but nobody was doing any hiring. Gent came over to the house and stayed with us until he got back.

When she walked in the door, Mama looked at her and said, "God, you poppin' sweat."

She said, "It feel like I'm 'bout to burn up."

"Here, lie down here on this chair in front of the fan."

THE FIRST CASE OF LUPUS

She put her hand on her forehead to see if she had a fever. She didn't feel warm. Then she felt her neck and rubbed her hand down her arm.

As she rubbed her arm, she said, "Lord, ya gettin' so little. What in the world wrong witcha?"

Gent didn't say anything. She just lay there with her eyes closed.

Then Mama lifted her blouse and felt her stomach.

"My God! You ain't hot nowhere but cha stomach! I'ma take ya to the doctor when Charlie get back. Where he gone?"

"Job huntin'," she said.

"Where else is there to go? He done been everywhere."

"I don't know."

"He might find somethin'. I hope so anyway."

"He said one time that he might go to the army. But I don't believe Charlie goin' to no army, not as hard as they say it is in there."

"Ya cooled off any yet?"

"Uh-huh, a little bit."

"Ya head ain't botherin' ya, is it?"

"A little but not too much."

"I be dog if we ain't got to find out what's wrong wit you. Essie be callin' to see how ya doin'. She asked me what was wrong witcha. I told her that I didn't know. She said that we should take ya off and have ya looked at."

"When?"

"She didn't say. I'ma take ya to the doctor first and see what he got to say 'bout it."

Mama went on in the kitchen, still talking to Gent. When she came back in the den, Gent had dosed off to sleep.

It was evening when Charlie got back. Gent was still on the chair, asleep.

He said, "How long she been here 'sleep?"

Mama said, "Ever since you left. She burnin' up wit a fever in her stomach. I wanted to take her to the doctor or the hospital, one."

"Well, we can go if ya ready. You gon' tell Randy?"

"No. He better not say nothin' 'bout me takin' that gal to the doctor."

On the way there, Charlie said, "Which one ya goin' to? Dr. Chad?"

"What time is it?" Gent asked him.

"Two thirty."

"Dr. Chad's office is closed. He won't be back till four."

Mama said, "Well, let's take her to the hospital then."

When they got her there, the emergency room doctor only checked her out a little, wrote her two prescriptions, and then released her. Gent came out mad and fussing. She walked right past Mama and Charlie without saying anything to them.

"What did the doctor say?" Mama asked.

"Nothin'. He didn't do nothin' but check ma temperature. I already knew that I had a fever. I coulda stayed home."

"What's that ya got in ya hand?"

"Just some dern prescriptions. I already got some of this medicine at the house. Let's go."

On the way back home, Mama told Charlie to stop at the store.

When she went into the store, he looked back at Gent and said, "I took the army test today."

"You kiddin'?"

"No, I ain't either. I couldn't find nobody that talked like they were doin' any hirin', so I took the test."

"I didn't think you was gonna do it. I thought you was bullshittin'."

"I told ya what I was gonna do. Next time, you'll believe me."

Mama got back in the car, and they told her about the army deal. She told them that, since the doctor didn't tell them anything, she was going to call Essie and let her know about what was going on.

Charlie and Gent got out at their house, and Mama drove the car home. Randy didn't even know that they were gone because he worked third shift and, when he went to sleep, it was hard to wake him up.

Mama told Aunt Kitty all about the hospital visit and how they didn't really do anything for her and that now they were going to try Aunt Essie's way. So they gave her a call.

THE FIRST CASE OF LUPUS

When she answered the phone, Mama said, "Hey, how ya doin'?"

"All right. Gent still havin' trouble wit her head?"

"Yeah. I had to take her to the hospital today. Her head was hurtin' her, and she had a fever."

"What did they say?"

"Nothin' much. I'ma take her back to the doctor in the mornin'."

"The doctor might not know what's wrong wit her. Somebody might have her fixed."

"Ain't no tellin', but they sho can't find out what's wrong wit her."

"I'm comin' home tomorrow and take her off. We'll find out what's wrong wit her one or another."

"All right. Where Kelly?"

"He gone wit Phil somewhere."

"He bringin' you down here, or you gon' drive yaself?"

"I'ma drive maself."

"Okay. I'll see ya tomorrow then."

"Okay, bye."

The next day, Aunt Essie was here early. Before eight, Mama was up and in the yards, working.

Aunt Essie asked Mama, "Ya ready to go?"

Mama said, "Yeah, just as soon as Gent get ready."

"Did ya tell her I was comin'?"

"Yeah. I told her after I got off the phone wit you last night."

A couple of minutes later, Gent walked up. "Hey," she said.

Aunt Essie turned around to her. "My God, you lost a lot of weight. You must ain't been eatin' nothin'?"

"I can't eat. I ain't got no appetite."

"Whatcha think caused that?"

"I don't know, Essie."

"Well, we gon' try to find out today."

They got in the car and left. They were on their way to Maxton, North Carolina, to see a witch doctor. On the way there, Gent told them that Charlie had taken the army test and passed it.

Essie said, "Army test? Is he gon' marry you before he go?"

"He ask me to, but not till he get out of basic trainin'."

"Why he gon' wait till then?"

"We thought it would be best if we wait and see where he gonna be stationed at first."

"Oh yeah, I see."

Mama said, "When all that happen? Last night?"

"No, he told me about it when you was in the store yesterday after we left the hospital. I mentioned it to ya when ya got back in the car, but you was talkin' 'bout Essie comin' today. When you came to the house last night, I meant to tell you then, but I forgot."

"This ain't gon' take too long, is it, Essie? I still wanna take her to the doctor. His office open at eleven."

"No. That's why I came early as I did."

When they got back, it was ten fifteen. Mama told Gent to go home and tell Charlie to get ready so they could go. When she got home, he was already dressed. They sat and talked for a minute. He asked her what happened.

She said, "Nothin' much. She gave me some old, bad-tastin' stuff to drink. Then we sat down at a table, and she read some cards. Don't ask me what they said 'cause I don't know. She said that somebody might have put somethin' down for Mama and I got it instead."

"Somethin' like what?"

"You know 'bout as much as I do. Then she said that a man had me fixed. To tell ya the truth, I don't believe nobody got nothin' like that on me."

"Essie believe in that stuff, don't she?"

"Shine yeah. That woman like to had me believin' it."

They heard Mama calling them.

Gent said, "We better go before Mama blood pressure go up."

"Yeah, we better."

When they got to Dr. Chad's office, Gent was poppin' sweat. Ever since it started getting warmer, she sweated like that. She always carried a hand towel with her to wipe her face. She wiped the sweat from her face as she signed her name on the list. Charlie asked her if she wanted him to sign it, but she said no and that she could do it.

THE FIRST CASE OF LUPUS

She went and sat where she could feel the air conditioner. When she sat down, she let out a breath of air like she had just walked ten miles.

Mama looked at her and said, "That little piece you had to walk got you that tired?"

"It ain't the walkin' that did it. It was climbin' them steps that got the best of me."

Then the nurse at the desk said, "Geneva, what is bothering you, hon?"

"I'm still havin' headaches, and my joints feel like they wanna get stiff on me."

"So it's about like the same thing you had before?"

"Yeah."

"All right, he'll be right with you in a minute."

A few minutes later, they called her back to be checked. She sat in the examining room waiting for him. Finally, he came in.

"Geneva, are you still having those headaches?"

"Yes, sir. They ease off, but they come right back. I have achin' in the joints too."

He examined her from head to toe. Then he started with the questions.

"I don't like this big change in your weight. When you were in the hospital in January, you weighed 125 pounds. Now you weigh only 95 pounds. How'd you lose so much weight, Geneva?"

"I ain't been eatin'. I just don't have no kinda appetite."

"How long has it been since you lost it?"

"Well, it started out to where I could eat about three or four spoonfuls of food each meal. Then some days, I couldn't eat nothin'. It went on like that for two or three weeks, and then it got to where I couldn't eat at all."

"Why didn't you tell me about your appetite the last time?"

"I was hopin' that I would get better without comin' here."

"I might have to put you back in the hospital. Your blood pressure is just a little high, but you have a high fever. We're going to have to do something about your eating problem."

"Well, if I go, do you think I'll be out by the first of the month? The guy I'm goin' to marry is leavin' in two weeks for basic trainin'."

"I'm not going to make any promises. If you go in this week, there is a chance you'll be out by then."

"Just what is it that you wanna have done?"

"I'm going to try and get that fever down and give you some glucose to give you some help with your blood system. Most of all, I want to do some tests to try and find out what's wrong with you. I'd be more concerned about getting better if I were you. That boyfriend of yours will be just fine if he knows that you're getting better."

"Well, I'll go 'cause I'm tired of feelin' the way I've felt these last few months. When do you want to start?"

"How does tomorrow morning sound?" he asked.

"Fine wit me. The sooner, the better."

"Good. I'll let them know that you'll be coming. I'll see you in the morning, Geneva."

"All right, thank you."

On the way back home, she told Mama and Charlie all about what the doctor had said. She told them that she didn't want to go back to the hospital because she wanted to see Charlie leave. He told her not to worry about seeing him off. If going to the hospital would help her any, she'd better go ahead.

When they pulled in the yard, Mama was the only one to get out. I ran to the door and asked them where they were going. They said uptown and told me to come and ride with them. That's when they told me about their plans and that Gent had to go back to the hospital again.

Gent said, "I sure hate to go."

Charlie said, "You goin'. You know that you're sick, so you better go and try to find out what's wrong witcha. 'Cause, you know, if anything happen to you and you go [die], I'll have to go too. Ain't that right, Head?"

I said, "Yeah, it must be love if you gon' die because she die."

We laughed.

When we got to town, we got out and went into the store. Gent got her some new panties and a pretty pink gown. Essie had given her the money for it. We went by Debra's house before we came home. As we pulled up in the yard, we could hear the music. She always played it loud. We got out of the car and went to the door. We had to knock hard for her to hear us, and we had to do it three or four times.

When she got to the door and opened it, she said, "I thought I heard somebody knockin'. Come on in. What's up?"

Gent said, "Nothin' much. I just came by to letcha know that I'm goin' to the hospital in the mornin'."

Charlie and I went in and sat down.

"Oh yeah? When you go to the doctor?"

"This mornin'. Girl, I don't weigh but ninety-five pounds."

"What! Girl, you lyin'?"

"I wish I was."

"Well, maybe this time they'll find out what's wrong witcha."

"I sho hope so. If I keep on like this, I'ma waste away to nothin', and I ain't got that much mo' to go."

"You ain't kiddin'. You losin' too fast."

Charlie said, "I told her old, stubborn ass to go to the doctor when Head showed me them pictures of her, but no, she kept puttin' it off."

She said, "Oh, you shut the hell up."

Charlie started laughing. We stayed a while longer and got high with Deb, then we got ready to go. We had to stop by the store for Mama.

When we got to the door Gent turned around and said to Deb, "Did Mama tell ya 'bout Charlie goin' in the army?"

"No. When?"

He said, "In two weeks."

Gent said, "That's why I don't want to go in the hospital yet. I want to go to the bus station with him when he leave."

"Well, you gotta see 'bout yaself first. You got to be able to go see him leave," Deb said.

"That's what I been tryin' to tell her," said Charlie.

"Well, I'll see ya later."

"Okay. Call me and let me know what room ya in."

"Okay."

I was leaving out behind Gent.

Deb said, "Silver Jean, you ought to stay and help me rake ma yards."

I said, "I would, but Mama want me to put down some rugs. She told me to do it before I left, but I told her I'd do it when I got back."

We got back to the house, and I started putting down the rugs. Gent and Charlie went home. She said that she wanted to get things together for her stay at the hospital.

The next morning, Mama, Gent, and Charlie got to the hospital at ten. They signed her in and put her in her room. They sat there and waited, but the doctor never came. At two, Charlie got up and told Mama that he was getting ready to go. She said okay and that, when the doctor came, she'd call home and tell him what he said.

He stayed at home and waited for the call. An hour later, the phone rang. I answered it. It was Mama.

"Hey, where everybody at?"

"Right here. Did you find out anything?"

"No. He looked at the x-rays, but he didn't find anything. Is Charlie there too?"

"Yes, ma'am."

"Let me speak to him."

I called him to the phone. He got on the phone.

"Yeah?"

"Hey, they didn't find anything."

"They didn't?"

"No. He said that he was gon' run some mo' test on her tomorrow and see what he can find."

"Is she 'sleep?"

"Yeah. She just dosed off not too long ago."

"Oh, let her sleep then."

"Let me speak to Kitty for a minute."

He handed her the phone.

"Hello."

"Hey, I'ma stay up here tonight. I wanna be here in the mornin' when the doctor come."

"Okay."

THE FIRST CASE OF LUPUS

"You called Essie?"

"Yeah. She said that she'd be back down here tonight."

Mama laughed and said okay and hung up the phone.

The next day, the nurse came by to take some blood for some tests. Dr. Chad had a list of different kinds of tests he wanted to do on her. He checked her for leukemia, cancer, sugar diabetes, and malaria. All the test came back negative. After he finished testing, he came in to see her.

"How you feeling today, Geneva?"

"About the same."

"I looked at the tests I have done on you, and I still couldn't find anything wrong with you."

"Well, I guess that should be good news, but it ain't."

"I know how you feel. But I'm going to keep trying."

He turned to leave, and Mama got up and went behind him.

When they got in the hall, Mama said, "Dr. Chad, is there somethin' that you ain't tellin' us?"

"I've told you all there is to tell. Your daughter isn't getting any better. All the test came back negative. To tell you the truth, Ms. Casey, I don't know what's wrong with her.

Naturally, Mama became upset and scared. "Whatcha mean you don't know? You're the doctor!"

"I'm sorry, Ms. Casey. I know you're hurting, but I've never seen anything like this before."

"All I know is that my gal is sick wit somethin'. You can tell that by lookin' at her. And you say that you don't know. Well, dammit, I'll find somebody that do."

He told her to go ahead and that sometimes a second opinion was the best thing. But in Gent's case, he didn't think that it was necessary.

She said, "You mighta gave up on her, but I sho ain't."

She went back in the room where Gent was.

"Dr. Chad couldn't find nothin' wrong witcha. I wanna get another doctor to look at cha. Is that all right wit you?"

"Yeah, if that's whatcha wanna do."

"We ain't got no choice. You can't go on like this. Which one do you wanna get?"

"I heard that Dr. Jason was a good doctor, but I don't know if he's takin' any new patients."

"I can tell the nurse to tell him to stop by here, and we can see. He can't say nothin' but yeah or no."

"Go head. I'm 'bout to worry myself to death not knowin' what's wrong wit me."

"Okay. I'll be right back." She went to the desk where the nurse was and asked her, "Will Dr. Jason be here any today?"

The nurse said, "Yes, ma'am. He should be here to make his rounds in about fifteen or twenty minutes."

"Could you please ask him to come by my daughter's room?"

"Yes, ma'am. What's your daughter's name and room number?"

"Geneva Casey. Room 122."

"All right, ma'am. I'll tell him as soon as he gets here."

"Thank you."

"You're welcome."

Mama went back in the room with Gent and waited for the doctor. Thirty minutes later, he came.

When he walked into the room, he said, "Hello, Ms. Casey, what can I do for you?"

Gent said, "I wanted to know if you was takin' any new patients? I need to get a second opinion."

"Who was your doctor before?"

"Dr. Chad," she said.

"What did he say was wrong with you?"

"He don't know. He couldn't find anything."

"I don't usually take a new patient unless I've checked them on an office visit first. But in your case, I'll make an exception."

"I sho thank you, Dr. Jason."

"I have to be honest with you. I'm doing it for myself as much as I'm doing it for you. I want to know what it is that Dr. Chad couldn't find. I'm not going to examine you until tomorrow. Right now, I want you to tell me about your illness."

THE FIRST CASE OF LUPUS

"At first, I started havin' headaches. They weren't too bad at first. I could take a Goody's Powder, and it would ease off. But then they started gettin' worse. I started takin' four Goody's instead of two. It got to where the Goody's Powders didn't do me any good. After the headaches, I lost ma appetite. Day after day, I ate less and less, then I just stopped eatin', period."

"When did the headaches begin?" he asked.

"In December."

"When did you go see your doctor?"

"Well, I was put in the hospital on New Year's Eve. Then the colder it got, ma leg joints started achin'. They felt like they wanted to get stiff. They bother me mostly when it's rainin' and cold. I have chills too."

"Is that all? I want you to tell me everything."

"Well, about a couple o' weeks ago, I got a fever. I went to Dr. Chad's to have it checked, and he said that it was pretty high."

Dr. Jason checked. "And he was right. Your temperature is 112, and we've got to get it down. I'll be back in the morning. I'm going to have the nurse give you something for the fever and have some tests on you starting first thing in the morning."

Mama said, "Dr. Chad run all kinds of test on her, and he didn't find anything wrong wit her."

"I'm going to check again. Maybe I'll see something he didn't."

"Oh, I see," said Mama.

He looked at Gent and said, "Geneva, how much did you weigh before you got sick?"

"A hundred and thirty-five pounds."

"And how much do you weigh now?"

"'Bout ninety or ninety-five pounds."

He quietly stood there for a few seconds and then left. The next morning, he had some tests done on her. That evening, when he looked at them, he couldn't find anything either. He did the same tests that Dr. Chad had done on her. He came by to examine her and to tell her about the test results.

"My test came back the same way Dr. Chad's did. Let me examine you right now. We'll talk about the tests after we finish. You'll have to wait in the hall, Ms. Casey."

Mama said all right and left. The nurse pulled the curtain between the beds, and Dr. Jason listened to her heartbeat. Then he checked her blood pressure. He said that it was up a little but not very much. He checked her temperature, and it had gone up one point.

"Geneva, this doesn't look very good. We have to get that fever down. I'm going to have one of the nurses bring in some medicine. Now, when you take it, drink plenty of water."

For two days, he tried to get the fever down. It would go down some but never back to normal.

He told Mama and Gent, "This is going to take a lot of time and patience for me to find out what it is that has her in this condition. I'm going to wait a couple of days before I can really get to work on you, Geneva. I'm going to get some things taken care of at the office, then I'll be back around to see you. Is that all right with you?"

"Well, I'd rather go home and wait them couple of days out with ma family, if I can."

"Sure, but you'll have to come back in a day or two."

"Okay," she said.

"All right, I'll release you, and I'll see you in a couple of days."

Dr. Jason left, and Gent called Charlie to come and pick them up. He was glad to hear that. He was at the hospital in no time. When they got home, Mama got on the phone and called Aunt Essie. Kelly answered the phone.

"Hey, where ya mama?"

"Right here." He called her on the phone.

"Hey, how ya doin'?" Mama asked.

"All right. How Gent doin'?"

"'Bout the same. Me and her talk to Dr. Jason today."

"You did? What did he say?"

"Nothin' much. 'Bout the same thing the other doctor said."

"Still don't know what's wrong wit her?"

"No."

"I mighta been right," said Essie.

"What?"

"Somebody got her fixed. Got somethin' on her. And the doctor ain't gon' find it if they is."

"Lord, I don't know."

"I'll be home tomorrow. We got to get some things straightened out. I meant to come back Tuesday, but I had some business to take care of."

"Child, that's all right."

"Well, I'ma go. I'll see ya tomorrow."

They said bye and hung up.

It was eight thirty the next morning when Kelly and Aunt Essie got to the house. Mama had cooked some grits, eggs, and sausage and was trying to get Gent to eat some.

Kelly said, "Nank, she shouldn't eat them eggs if she got a fever."

"Why come?" Mama said.

"They told us in the army that, if a person got fever, they shouldn't have stuff like milk, grits, or eggs 'cause it'll only make it worse."

"Oh, I didn't know that. I can't get her to eat it anyway."

"The best thing to give her is some juice or fruit."

Aunt Essie took some money out of her pocketbook and told Kelly, "Here, go get her some."

Kelly took the money and told Randy to ride with him.

Essie said, "No, you better go by yo'self. If Randy go, you'll never get back, and I got somewhere to go."

Randy said, "Ah, woman, you ain't got nowhere to go this time of the mornin'."

"Yes, I is to."

Randy said, "Come on, Kelly. We comin' right back."

They stayed gone for about an hour.

Essie said, "I knowed they won't comin' right back."

Mama said, "Where you got to go?"

"Off a piece. Me and Gent got to take a ride."

Gent said, "Where we suppose to be goin'?"

"To see a woman 'bout somethin'," she said.

"Ah, come on now, Essie. I ain't up for a whole lotta ridin' now."

"It ain't a whole lot. It ain't that far."

When Kelly and Randy got back, they left. They stayed gone for hours. I kept saying to myself that Gent was mad. When they got back, it was four. When Gent got out of the car, she didn't say anything to anybody. She just went into the house with a frown on her face.

Essie came up on the porch after her, saying, "Oh yeah, we got our stuff together. Everything gon' be all right."

I went into the room where Gent was. She told me all about what went on.

I said, "What happened this time?"

She said, "Girl, you ain't gonna believe this. She took me back to the same one, and she did 'bout the same thing she did the last time. But this time, she wanted me to stay there until dark so that we could go to the graveyard, but I told Essie that I was feelin' bad and I wanted to go home and lie down. That's the only reason she left 'cause she was gonna stay if I hadn't said nothin'."

"What did she give ya to drink this time?"

"Girl, she gave me a whole jar of somethin'. I think it's that same stuff she gave me the first time."

"And you gonna drink it?" I asked.

"Yeah. I don't wanna hurt Essie's feelin's."

I looked at her with disbelief. I couldn't believe she was going to drink that stuff. I didn't believe in it, but Essie did faithfully. I was really scared of the stuff.

Charlie came in the room and told her that they had to talk. He told her that he had received a letter from the array saying that he had to be there Monday morning.

She said, "You can't change ya mind now."

"I know that," he said. "I sho hate to leave ya like this. I don't know if I can make it six weeks in basic if I leave ya as sick as ya is now. I'll probably go crazy over there."

"Don't worry 'bout me. If anything happens, I can call and letcha know."

"That's just what I mean. Being that you ain't my wife, if anything do happen to ya, they might not let me come home. They try to be tough about things like that."

"I know. Maybe nothin' won't happen. I hope not anyway."

"Me either. Whatcha think we should do?"

"Whatcha mean?" she asked.

"Do ya wanna get married before I go, or do ya still wanna wait till I finish basics?"

"We can wait. I think it'll be better."

"Why ya say that?"

"Because we don't know if I'm goin' to get any better or not. Maybe, by the time you come back from trainin', I'll be doin' a little better." Then she said in a low voice, "Or dead, one."

"Well, if that's whatcha want."

Then Essie walked in. "Charlie, I wanna talk to ya when ya get time," she said.

Charlie said okay, and she left.

He looked at Gent and said, "I wonder what she wants to talk to me about?"

Gent said, "Ain't no tellin', but go and see what she want anyway."

"I am. I'll be back to letcha know."

He went out on the porch and asked her what it was she wanted to talk to him about. She told him to walk around the house with her.

When they got 'round there, she said, "You still gon' wait till ya get back from the army before y'all get married?"

"Yep, she said that she'd rather wait."

"How come? From the way things look, she might not be here when you get back."

Charlie stood there for a while and was quiet. Then he said, "Well, she said that she wanted to wait."

"Well, you need to talk to her and see if you can change her mind. I'ma talk to her 'cause I don't think y'all should wait."

"I don't really want to wait either, but she do," he said.

"I'ma talk to her and see what she say. I'll letcha know somethin' when I finish."

Charlie said okay, and Essie went into the house. She went right to the room where Gent was. She told Gent all about how she shouldn't wait to get married and that Charlie loved her. She said that, if he wanted to marry her, she ought to go ahead because she might not get that chance again. Essie gave a little laugh and said that, if she was Charlie, she sure wouldn't marry her. Instead, she'd be out trying to find somebody else. He was proving his love to her by asking her to be his wife. She got up to leave and looked back at Gent and told her to think about what she said.

Gent said, "Okay, but I still rather wait."

Essie went back outside and told Charlie to go into the room where she was.

When he walked in, Gent said, "What you back so soon for? Essie been talkin' to ya and gotcha scared?"

He laughed and said, "Yep. She told me that, if we didn't get married before I went in the army, cha might not be here when I get back."

She laughed and said, "Whatcha think we should do?"

"Well, what she said makes a lot of sense. The main reason I don't wanna wait is that you're so sick."

They decided to go on and do it.

When they told us that they were going to, Aunt Essie said, "I knowed y'all would see it ray 'way. Now we gotta tell everybody about it."

Mama said, "When y'all plannin' on doin' it?"

Charlie said, "Gent wanna do it on Ricky's birthday."

"When is that?" asked Mama.

"The twenty-seventh of this month."

I looked at the calendar and said, "That's this Saturday. Today's date is the twenty-third."

Na and Randy started picking at her, saying that they had a good reason to get drunk this weekend. Na said that this was something he had to see because he thought that the bummer (Gent) would never get married, and everybody started laughing.

THE FIRST CASE OF LUPUS

Mama wasn't very happy about the news because she didn't want her to get married, not with her being as sick as she was. It hurt her even more when Charlie said that he was going to send for her after he got stationed.

Aunt Kitty and Mama called everybody and told them the news about Gent and Charlie.

It came as a surprise to them, and just about everybody they told said, "My God, he must really love that girl to wanna marry her in the shape she's in."

When they called Aunt Clovis and Uncle Thomas to tell them, Gent wanted to speak to Quandra. Aunt Clovis said that she wasn't there, but she'd tell her to call her as soon as she got there. She and Mama talked for a while and then hung up.

At six, Quandra called back. Sterling answered the phone.

"Hi, Sterling, how you doin'?"

"All right."

"Where's Gent?"

"Right here. Just a minute, I'll get her." He put the phone next to the chair she was sitting in.

She said, "Hello."

"Hi, girl. How ya doin'?"

"Pretty good, I reckon. How you doin'?"

"I'm okay."

"Did Aunt Clovis tell ya the news about me and Charlie?"

"Yeah. Congratulations. I'm glad you left word for me to call ya back. I have some news of my own, but I want you to keep it a secret because I haven't told Mama yet."

"Okay. What is it?"

"Ricky and I are planning on getting married again."

"Oh yeah! I'm glad for ya. I know Head'll be glad to hear that," said Gent.

"Yeah, we're talking about tying that knot again. How do you feel about a double weddin'?" Quandra asked.

"That sounds good to me."

"You'll have to ask Charlie and see how he feel about it, don't cha?"

"No. As long as we get married, it don't matter. The reason I wanted to talk to you was to see if maybe you had a dress or a gown that's too small for you that I could borrow."

"I believe I do. Mama didn't tell me when y'all were going to do it. So when is the big day?"

"Saturday, the twenty-seventh."

"What time, or do it depend on what time you get there?"

"I'm hopin' it'll be around two or three. I sho hope we don't have to wait too long 'cause, when I sit up too long, I start feelin' bad."

"I hope so too for yo' sake. I'm not gonna tell Mama and Daddy about me and Ricky until we get ready to go down there Saturday."

"You know she gon' have a damn fit."

"I know. I don't think that Daddy will mind too much, just as long as it's what I want."

"He might not, but Clovis sho is."

"You ain't wrong, coz. I hate to tell her, but she's gonna have to know before the time come."

"I'm glad I ain't the one that got to tell her."

"And I wish that I didn't."

Gent said, "Well, cuz, I'ma letcha go and do whatcha gotta do, and I'll see ya Saturday."

"I might be home before then to help get some things for a reception afterward."

"All right, I'll see ya then. Love ya. Bye-bye."

Cille, our next-door neighbor, was coming over to see Gent just as she was hanging up the phone. She sat in the chair next to Gent.

Cille said, "I hear that y'all gettin' ready to do that thing."

Charlie was coming out the kitchen with his plate and said, "Yep."

"I hear ya. I didn't think you'd ever get married, girl, but when Charlie came and hooked ya, you just couldn't pass 'em up."

Charlie said, "That's right. She know what's good for her."

"Shit, you know what's good for you too," Gent said.

We laughed.

Cille said, "I know Essie comin' to it, ain't she?"

THE FIRST CASE OF LUPUS

Mama said, "Whatcha mean comin'? She ain't never went nowhere."

"Ya mean she been down here all this time?"

"If she go home, she come back the same day. She said, as long as Gent's sick, she'll be right here."

Gent said, "I know there was somethin' I meant to tell y'all. Guess who else is gettin' married?"

All of us said, "Who?"

"Quandra and Ricky."

Mama said, "Gal, you lyin'?"

"No, I ain't either."

"Oh, I know Clovis is havin' a fit," said Cille.

"No, she ain't 'cause she don't know it yet. She said that she won't gon' tell her till Saturday right before she come down here."

"Oh, Lord, she gon' come in raisin' hell," said Mama.

"Yep," Gent said.

"What they get a divorce for if they knew that they still loved each other?"

"I don't know, but they sho gon' tie the knot again."

Charlie said, "They gon' get married the same day we do?"

"Yep, and the same time."

Cille said, "What, a double weddin'? There ain't no sign in that Nank?"

"No, not that I know of."

"A double weddin'. That should be nice," Charlie said.

"She said that she'll be here before Saturday because she wanna get some stuff for a reception. You gon' cook the cake, Mama?"

"What kind do ya want?"

"It don't matter. What kind do ya think would be best?"

"I'd better not cook a layer cake 'cause that won't last no time, so I better make a sheet cake."

"That'll be good enough. That way, everybody can get a piece."

Mama asked Charlie, "Did ya call ya mama and daddy and tell them?"

"Yes, ma'am."

"Well, ya better call again and tell ya brothers and sisters about the reception."

He got up and went to call. He didn't stay in the room long before he was back out. Gent thought that he didn't get an answer.

She said, "Won't nobody home?"

"Yeah, there was somebody there. I told Pat, and she gon' tell the rest of 'em."

"Do ya think they'll come?" Gent asked him.

"Yeah, the kids'll come, but I don't know 'bout Mama and Daddy."

Mama said, "Well, we'll just send them a plate then."

"Ya told Tom and Frank?"

"I ain't seen 'em nowhere to tell 'em."

Charlie spent that night at his parents' house. Joe Ward called to see how Gent was doing. He wanted to come and see her, but he was scared. He had heard some talk about us being mad at him because we thought he had put roots (a hex) on Gent. Mama told him that, that wasn't true and, if he wanted to come and see Gent, to come on because no one was mad at him. He said that he didn't know for sure and that that's why he hadn't been around. We knew better than that. He hadn't been around because he hit Ella at the club that night and he was scared to face Kelly or Essie. They got that settled, and Mama gave Gent the phone.

She said, "Hello."

"How ya doin'?" he asked.

"I'll make it, I reckon. How you doin'?"

"All right. When can I come and see ya?"

"You can come whenever ya want to. I'm gettin' married this weekend."

"Whatcha wanna go and do somethin' like that for? Ya sure that's whatcha want?"

"Yep."

"Ya don't love 'em, so whatcha marryin' him for? I can take care of ya if that's whatcha want."

"How ya figure I don't love him? I wouldn't marry him if I didn't."

THE FIRST CASE OF LUPUS

"Don't do it, please. I'm beggin' ya. Don't do it."

"Ma mind's made up. This time Saturday, I'll be a married woman."

"Well, there ain't nothin' I can say to change ya mind. I hope ya be happy. I reckon I'll see ya later. You'll always be my favorite." Then he hung up.

Joe knew the reason Gent broke up with him is that he cheated on her with another woman. That's why she and Charlie went together in the first place; it was because of his wrongdoing.

Everything was happening so fast. They had to plan a wedding for Saturday. Charlie had to report for duty on Monday, and she had to go back to the hospital on the same day he had to leave.

Cille came to sit and spend some time with Gent, but she didn't want to keep her up if she wanted to lie down and get some rest. So she asked her before she made herself comfortable.

"Yeah, I'm sure. Sit down and talk awhile."

She sat in the chair next to the bed. "I hope the Fayetteville crowd don't spoil things for ya."

"I don't either 'cause I sho don't feel up to bearin' a whole lotta noise today."

It seemed like Saturday came so fast.

"I know whatcha mean, especially with ya head botherin' ya the way it is."

"Did ya tell Tim that I was gettin' married today?"

"Yeah, he said that he won't comin' to see you no mo' till Charlie leave 'cause you know he was yo' boyfriend. Lord, that boy tickled me."

"That's why he ain't been to see me yet? He come and see me every day."

"Yeah, he mad witcha."

Then we heard Mama in the kitchen.

"Oh, Lord, here we go."

I said, "She look like she steamin' too."

Cille got up and went in the den and looked out the window. "Oh, she pissed off. She got her bottle though."

43

They got here before Quandra and Ricky did, and when she came in, she was fussing.

"I swear I could kill that damn Quandra."

Uncle Thomas said, "If she happy with him, let her have him, long as she's happy."

He was already feeling pretty good when he got here, but he still wanted to give a toast to the brides and grooms. When Charlie came over to the house, Uncle Thomas asked him to have one with him.

Then he looked at Aunt Clovis and said, "Be happy for ya baby, sis."

The whole time he talked, she looked at him while rolling her eyes.

Then she said in a snappy way, "Oh, just shut the hell up to me, Thomas. You don't care about yo' own ass, so just shut up to me."

He looked over at Mama and said, "Am I right, sis?"

Mama said, "Yeah, you sho is."

"But, Nank, he ain't got nothin' to offer her but his Black ass," said Aunt Clovis.

"Well, I ain't never had one to give me nothin'. That's why I ain't got no husband."

Aunt Clovis got up and went into the room where Gent was. "Hey, baby, how you doin'? 'Bout the same?" she asked.

"I feel so-so, but I'm hangin' in there."

"Well, thank the Lord for that."

"I do, every day."

"What time is the weddings gonna start?"

"We have to be there at two."

"Y'all got a while to wait."

"Tell ya the truth, I'm ready to get it over with. I feel so bad."

"Well, stay in bed until 'bout time to go. I'll help Nank getcha ready."

"All right, I won't plannin' on gettin' up now anyway."

"When did Quandra tell you about her and Ricky?"

"The same day that Mama called and told you about me and Charlie. But she told me that night when she called me back."

THE FIRST CASE OF LUPUS

"And didn't say nothin' to me about it until this mornin'. I felt like chokin' that girl when she told me that shit," said Aunt Clovis.

"She said that they had been thinkin' about it for a good while."

"I didn't say nothin' to her this mornin' because I was too mad, but after all this is over with, I'ma have a long talk with that sister."

She left and went back to the den where Mama and Aunt Kitty were. She was mad for the rest of the day. She hardly said anything to anyone, but Essie didn't care. She thrived on making a situation worse.

When Quandra and Ricky came, she didn't say anything to either one of them. She was on the porch when they drove up.

I went to the car to meet them. "Hi, cousins."

"Hey, cuz," they said.

"Where is everybody?" asked Quandra.

"In the house."

We went into the room where Gent was.

Quandra said, "Hi, Gent. How ya doin'? Let me get some sugar." She kissed her on the cheek.

"I'm livin'. Thank God for that."

"Where's Charlie?"

"He went uptown for somethin'."

Then Ricky walked in. "Hey, sweets, how ya doin'?"

"All right. Look like you feelin' good."

"I am. Where ya brothers at?"

"Na went to see a woman, and Randy went to take Charlie uptown."

"I got some good shit I want him to try."

"He should be back in a few minutes."

"Oh, I ain't goin' nowhere," he said.

Quandra and Ricky were already dressed when they got here. When Charlie got back, it was after one. He had to hurry and get ready. Gent had more than enough help getting dressed. Mama and Aunt Kitty were doing one thing, and Essie and Aunt Clovis were doing another. Essie fixed her hair, and for her to be as sick as she was, they had her looking pretty good.

Na went and got dressed in a hurry. He said that this was one wedding he didn't wanna miss. He and Randy couldn't believe that Gent was finally tying the knot.

Cille kept saying, "You always said you won't gon' get married. What happened?"

They all got ready to go. Mama went into her room and lay across the bed and cried as Gent went out the door. Na rode with Aunt Clovis and Uncle Thomas, and the brides and grooms rode together. Na took a picture of them as they were getting in the car, and right then and there, I and Cille decided to get some film and take some too.

While they were at the chapel, we were running around town trying to find film; and finally, we did. We went back to get a picture of them coming out the door, but they were already gone. We circled the block and caught up with them on Main Street. They were blowing their horns, so when we caught up with them, we blew ours too.

When we got to the house, the few people we had invited were waiting in the yard. We got out when we parked and asked the guests if there was anything we could get for them. Gent and Cille were standing in the front yard talking.

Cille said, "Y'all sho didn't stay in there long. Me and Silver Jean went to get some film, and when we got back, y'all was gone."

"Yeah, they got us as soon as we signed the license. They said that I didn't look like I was feelin' too good, so they let us go on in."

"That was good. Well, how ya feel now?"

"Bad. Feel like I'm sick on the stomach. I believe I'll go lie down for a while. Maybe I'll feel a little better."

"I'll walk in witcha. Want me to help ya in the house?"

"No. I think I can make it."

When they came in, Mama asked her, "Whatcha gettin' ready to do? Sit down awhile?"

She said, "No, ma'am. I'ma go to bed. I don't feel like sittin' up right now."

Cille stayed in the room for a while with her, talking about the future. When Gent dozed off, she came back outside and started celebrating with the rest of us. We tried the reefer Ricky had, and it

THE FIRST CASE OF LUPUS

was good. We stayed in the yard for a long time getting high. Then Aunt Clovis sent for Quandra so that they could have their little discussion. Essie was running from house to house trying to find Gent something to wear on her honeymoon.

Mama didn't think that she should go. "That gal ain't goin' on no honeymoon, sick as she is. You oughta know better than that."

Essie said, "Why not? She gon' have her husband wit her if anything should happen."

"I know that. That ain't got nothin' to do wit it. Charlie ain't got no money for no motel room."

"Yes, he is."

"Where he get it from?"

"Me."

"It's up to Gent. If she wanna go, she can go."

"I know she can."

Mama just sucked her teeth and walked off. She knew there wasn't any use in fussing with Essie because she was going to do what she wanted to anyway. She didn't say another word. They got her spoiled like that because she's the baby of fifteen kids.

Charlie went home to change and told Mama that he'd be right back. She went back and looked in on Gent. When she pulled the curtain back, Gent turned and looked at her.

"I thought you was sleep."

"I was, but Aunt Clovis and Quandra woke me up wit their talk."

"Charlie went home to change clothes. He said he'll be right back."

"What Essie doin'?"

"In there gettin' you somethin' to take to the motel."

"I didn't know that I was goin' to a motel."

"That's what she said. She gave Charlie the money. You don't feel like goin', do ya?"

"No, but I'll go. I don't wanna hurt Essie's feelin's."

"How long they been 'round there?"

"Who?" asked Gent.

"Clovis and Quandra."

47

"I don't know, but she talkin' shit about her marryin' Ricky again."

"She oughta gone and leave that girl alone. She gotta live her own life. Well, ya know ya ain't gotta go. Call me in the mornin', and I'll have Na or Randy pick y'all up."

"Okay. Is Essie 'bout got ma stuff ready?"

"I believe she is. Let me go see."

Before Mama could make it to the door, Charlie met her with the suitcase in his hand. Quandra was behind him.

"We're on our way out, cuz. Do ya want me to drop y'all off at the room? Essie said somethin' about y'all goin'," Quandra said.

"Yeah. She said that she was gonna tell Kelly to take us, so ya better tell him that we gonna catch y'all."

"Okay. Give me ya suitcase so I can put it in the trunk."

Charlie said, "I'll take it. I gotta go to the house for somethin' anyway."

"All right, I'm ready anytime you are."

"Well, I'm comin' on out. We can pick Charlie up from the house."

"All right. Aunt Nank, I'll probably see you next weekend."

"Okay, baby, take care."

"You too."

"I will."

Then Ricky came back in and said to me, "You gonna come and spend some of the summer wit us?"

"I'll letcha know, cuz, but ain't no tellin' I might."

"All right, you do that. Bye, Aunt Nank. Oh yeah, I left ya one on ya dresser. See ya later."

They left.

The next morning, Gent called for somebody to get them at nine thirty.

"Where Mama at?" she said.

"In her room. Hold on. I'll get her."

I went into the room to tell her that Gent was on the phone, but she had already picked it up before I got there.

"Hey, you ready to come home?"

THE FIRST CASE OF LUPUS

"Yes, ma'am. You can tell whoever's comin' to come on."

"All right, I'ma send him on."

She went into the room and woke up Randy. She had to call him a few times, but she finally got him up. He got up with a pout and a frown on his face. He asked Mama which motel were they in, and then he left.

I got their room ready and fixed Gent's chair for her. Mama gave them the boys' room because it was the only one that had a door to it. Since Charlie was leaving to go in the army, Mama told them it would be best if she moved back home with us because she didn't want her staying by herself.

When she got home, we sat in the den and talked for a long time. I was anxious to find out how her honeymoon went. So I asked her.

"Girl, it won't good at all. I felt so sick on the stomach all night. Charlie walked over to a gas station and brought me a Alka-Seltzer. I drunk that and went to sleep. Over in the night, I woke up wit a headache, and he had to go back again for some Goody's powders."

"You didn't enjoy yo'self none then, did ya?"

"Not a bit."

"Sound like I hear Debra Jean comin'."

"It is. I see her comin' by Mr. Plana's house."

We were just finishing the joint Ricky had left for me the day before. Mama didn't want Gent to smoke, but she did anyway. Mama was on the porch when Deb came up.

"Hey, Mama. Where everybody at?" Debra asked.

"They in there smokin' that shit," she said.

"Gent in there too?"

"Yeah, she in there wit the crowd. If she ate as much as she smoke that shit, she'd be all right."

Deb laughed and walked into the house. "What's happenin'?"

We said, "Nothin' much."

"This all y'all newlyweds got to do?"

Gent said, "Yep, this is about it."

Deb looked at me. "Y'all gotta game today?"

"Yeah, we play Little Rock."

"I might go to that game, Ma and Bern."

Berniece was her sister-in-law, and they hung together all the time.

I left at three to go play ball. We beat by nine runs. When I got home, Gent was still waiting in the den to ask me who won.

"We did, 11 to 20."

"Hear ya. How many games y'all lost so far?"

"One."

"I sho miss goin' to see y'all play."

"And we miss yo' mouth too."

She laughed a little. "Well, I reckon I'll go lie down. This chair got ma butt hurtin'."

Mama picked at her. "What butt? You ain't got none."

"I got 'bout as much as you got. Charlie love it even if it ain't much."

We laughed, and they went on in their room.

Aunt Hannah came by to see Gent. She was just leaving church, and she had Mr. Mun and Mrs. Viola to bring her by there. Mama saw them coming up in the yard, so she met them at the door.

"Hey, Nank. Where ma girl at?" Aunt Hannah asked.

"She 'round there in the room. How y'all doin'? Come on in."

"Just fine. How you doin'?"

"I'm makin' it wit the help of the Lord."

"I come by to say a prayer for ma girl."

"She 'round there in the room. Just go right behind, Hannah."

Aunt Hannah said to Gent, "I bought Mr. Mun by to pray for ya. Do ya feel up to it?"

"Yes, ma'am. I ain't gon' never turn down a prayer."

"Go in the den where there's enough room," said Mama.

Gent got up, and they went and got started. Aunt Hannah played the piano after they finished praying. They stayed for an hour or more.

When he got ready to leave, Gent said, "Will you please and pray for me again when you ain't too busy?"

I could tell that it made Mr. Mun feel good to hear her say that. He said, "Yes, I sho will."

THE FIRST CASE OF LUPUS

"It made me feel so good. Like everything was gonna be all right."

Aunt Hannah got happy and started shoutin'. Then Mama started playing the piano.

After she calmed down, Gent said, "Aunt Hanna, you make sure thatcha bring him back now."

"Don't worry, I will. Mr. Mun, you 'bout ready to go? I got a program to play today."

"Yeah, but I will be back."

"Thank you. I'll be lookin' for ya. Yo' prayer sho have done somethin' for me. I'll never forget it."

"God bless ya, child," he said, and they left.

Later that evening, Gent started feeling worse and told Mama that she had to take her somewhere. She said that she couldn't hardly rest anywhere she got. She said that she didn't understand how she could feel so bad now as good as she felt this evening when Aunt Hannah and the Johnsons were there. Mama told Charlie to help her get ready, and they took her to the hospital.

They were on their way to St. Eugene, but Mama told him to go to Marion Hospital instead. When they got her there, they examined her and found she had hemorrhoid trouble. They sent her home and said, if she got any worse, to bring her back. The next day, they did just that. This time, they kept her. She had to stay for two weeks.

Mama and Charlie called Dr. Jason's office and told him that she couldn't make it back and told him why. He said that he understood and that he could use the extra time to finish what he had to do. He said he'd call when he thought she was back home.

Charlie had to leave for basic training on the one o'clock bus. Gent was feeling so bad that she didn't even think about him leaving.

Two days after Gent went to the hospital, Cille wanted me to take her to put in an application. She said that she was tired of sitting around home doing nothing. We went to a few places in town where she thought they might be hiring. Then she decided that she wanted to go to the Heritage plant in Marion. Right before we got to the hospital, the car backfired and shot out black smoke. Then we coasted a little way over, and it died.

Cille said, "Ain't this somethin'? Time we get to the hospital, the car cuts off. Gent must know that we won't comin' by to see her."

"You ain't kiddin'," I said.

"I'ma call Bopete and tell him about this car. While we waitin' on him, we'll go see Gent."

"Okay."

"I'ma tell her about where the car tore up on us at too."

"I know she gon' pick at us," I said.

"Yeah. We won't plannin' on doin' nothin' but puttin' in an application."

"That's why she gonna pick, 'cause we won't comin' to see her."

We went to the front desk and got some passes to her room.

When we got there, I asked her, "Where Mama at?"

Before she could answer, Mama was coming out the bathroom. She said to Cille, "I thought you was job huntin'?"

"I am. The car tore up right down the road from here before we got to the hospital."

I said, "Cille said that Gent felt us gettin' ready to go on past here without stoppin', so she wished us bad luck."

Gent smiled but didn't say anything. She didn't have much to say, period. Cille and I talked to Mama for a few minutes and then left. By the time we got back to the car, Bopete was there.

Cille looked at me in a funny way and said, "It sure seem like he got here quick, don't it?"

"Yeah, or we was gone a long time one."

He went under the hood and then got in the car and turned the key, and it started right up. I took her to fill out her application, and then we came back home.

The next week on a Tuesday, they brought her home.

She told Mama to put her back in the boys' room. She said that she could rest better in there than she could in her room, so Mama said okay.

The nights were getting longer and longer for Mama.

She hardly rested at night. She always listened for anything happening to Gent. She told Aunt Kitty that, whenever Gent lay down

THE FIRST CASE OF LUPUS

at night to sleep, she didn't know if she was going to wake up to see another day.

Aunt Kitty told Mama that she shouldn't think like that and that, if she kept worrying herself like that, she'd be gone before Gent was. All Mama would say was that she couldn't help it and that it was a mother's place to worry about her kids.

The way Gent breathed it sounded like each breath was her last one. Sometimes I'd walk in the room where she was, and she'd be lying in the bed talking to God.

"Lord, I can't suffer like this too much longer. I thank you for keepin' me here this long, but, Lord, I'm tired of sufferin' like this."

Randy came into the room and asked her if she wanted him to put her stereo in the room with her. She said yes. He went into his room, which was Aunt Kitty's old room, and got it. As soon as he put it down, she told him to get her record and put it on. He got on the other bed in the room and listened to it with her. He lit up a joint.

"If this smoke is botherin' you, I'll put it out," he said.

She said, "No. Go on and smoke it. It don't bother me until I try to smoke it. I'm tryin' to kick the habit."

So he smoked it alone.

The following Monday, Dr. Jason's office called and said for her to come by the office about ten thirty that morning. Mama and I took her. He asked her what happened in Marion and wanted to know if they had found out anything.

She told him, and she said no and that they hadn't found anything. He said she needed to be ready to go back to the hospital the next morning.

"I'm glad to hear that. This time, ya might find out what's wrong with me. I'm hopin' so anyway."

"I might. Let's hope so," he said.

On the way back home, Mama asked her, "When ya gon' tell the welfare people thatcha got married?"

"After Charlie get out of basic trainin'."

"When is that?"

"About three or four mo' weeks."

"Well, maybe they won't find out nothin' before then. I hope not anyway."

"Me either," said Gent.

The next day, she was admitted to the hospital. Mama stayed with her all day. When Cookie and I walked in, she was standing up getting ready to go.

"How y'all get here?" Gent said.

"We caught a ride wit Tom," I said.

"Is Bobby Gene comin' to pick ya up?"

"I don't know. I'ma have to call and see. If he don't, I'll have to wait till somebody come up here."

Mama said, "Y'all can stay here till I come back. I got to go pick up Essie. She gonna come and stay all night."

"Let me check wit him first."

I called. He said that he would come, so I told her to go ahead. We talked with Gent for a long time before Aunt Essie came. But when Essie did, she started talking as soon as she hit the door.

"The doctor been by yet?"

"Not yet," Gent said.

Then she looked at me and said, "How you goin' home? Bobby Gene?"

"Yes, ma'am."

"I didn't know y'all was gonna be up here."

"Mama knew. We was here when she left to go getcha."

"Oh," she said and took a brown paper bag out of her pocketbook and put it in the drawer next to Gent's bed.

She looked at Gent and said, "This the stuff. Nank wouldn't bring it, so I brought it maself."

Gent thought sure that she was through with that stuff. She had a frown on her face.

Essie said, "I know ya don't like it, butcha gotta take it like ya been doin'."

"Well, if ya gon' put it in there, wrap it in a towel so nobody won't see it."

"Yeah, 'cause I don't want 'em to know ya got it."

Next she pulled out a pair of pink bedroom slippers.

THE FIRST CASE OF LUPUS

She looked at me and Cookie and said, "I don't wanna catch y'all feet in 'em."

I said, "I ain't got no business up here wit no bed slippers on."

"I ain't talkin' 'bout up here. I'm talkin' 'bout when she get home."

"We don't wear 'em there either," said Cookie.

We stayed a little longer before Bobby came. Instead of calling on the phone for me, he came to the room to see how Gent was doing. Then we left.

Mama went back the next day, but she wasn't in her room when she got there. Dr. Jason had them to take her down for more x-rays. Again they came back negative. Her fever was steadily rising. When she got back to her room, she told them that, while she was in the lab, they weighed her. When Mama asked her how much she weighed, she said seventy-seven pounds. Mama didn't want to believe it. Essie just stood there, shaking her head.

She said, "They ain't gon' find nothin' wrong wit her because somebody got her rooted. Just as sho as I'm sittin' here in this chair. I know what I'm talkin' 'bout."

Mama sucked her teeth and turned her head. She told Essie that she was going to stay and that she could go home with the car. She stayed a little while longer and then left. She told Mama to call if she found out anything.

Dr. Jason came by early the next day. He told her that he wanted to take some bone marrow from her leg. He took it with a long needle. They put her to sleep when he did it because of the pain. Those tests were negative too. After examining the results, he came back to talk to Mama and Gent.

He said, "I don't know exactly what I'm looking for, but I haven't found anything yet. If I'm going to find it, it'll have to be soon because she's slipping away from us more and more each day."

Mama asked, "Whatcha gonna do now?"

"I'm not giving up yet. I'm going to call a doctor overseas. I'll tell him all of her symptoms, how they started, and hopefully he'll have some idea of what it is."

"I hope to God y'all can come up wit somethin'."

"I'm going to do my best."

"Oh, I know ya will."

"Meanwhile, y'all pray, and I'll pray. Between us and the good Lord, something's bound to happen."

"Well, I been doin' that all the time, ever since she been this way, and I ain't 'bout to stop now."

Gent lay there without saying a word.

"All right, Ms. Casey. I'll see you in the morning after I talk to the doctor."

A nurse came by a few minutes later to give her some pain medicine.

Mama asked her, "Will Dr. Jason be by the same time tomorrow as he did today?"

"Yes, ma'am. She's his only patient for a while. He turned the rest of his patients over to Dr. Stan for the time being."

"Oh, I didn't know that. Thank you."

The nurse left.

Mama looked at Gent and said, "That man mean business, don't he? Maybe we shoulda been had him."

Gent said, "You ain't kiddin'. I'd probably been out of here by now if we had."

"Lord, I hope he find out what's wrong witcha."

"I sho hope so."

Later in the night, Gent started complaining about pain in the leg they had taken the marrow from. Mama pushed the button for the nurse to come and give her something for it. She came to the room, and Mama told her what the problem was. She told Mama that she'd have to check with the doctor before she could give her anything. Mama thought that she would have to wait till the next day before she could get anything, but she didn't. The nurse then told her that she would call him and see what he said. She left and returned quickly. When she walked back into the room, Gent was lying still with her eyes closed and moaning.

The nurse had three long capsules in a cup. She put her arm around Gent's neck to help her sit up and take her medicine. After she took it, she dozed off. Mama sat in the chair next to her bed,

THE FIRST CASE OF LUPUS

looking at Gent. She had lost so much weight that her cheekbones were clearly visible.

Her eyes had fear in them and little hope. The worst was yet to come.

Dr. Jason came by the next morning. "Good morning, Geneva. How's that leg?"

"It's okay. It don't hurt as much as it did last night."

"That's good. Did the medicine help much?"

"Yes, sir. It put me to sleep."

"Well, that's exactly what I wanted it to do."

She asked him, "How did everything go with that doctor?"

"I'm glad you asked. I found out what it is you have. It's a blood disease called lupus. I'm going to be honest with you. There is no cure for this disease, and in your case, it's too far gone to be treated. If you overcome this, it will be a miracle. If you would try to eat something, you'd be helping yourself a lot. Even three or four spoonfuls a day will help."

She said, "I try to eat, but I can't no matter how hard I try."

"Pray and ask the Lord to help you, Geneva. The way the fever has cooked your mouth, I think it would be best if you stopped smoking."

"I will. It hurts when I smoke anyway."

Mama said, "Can I take her home?"

He motioned his head for her to go into the hall.

"Yes, you can take her home, but to tell you the truth, I think it would be easier for you and your family if you'd put her in a home. With this disease, she's not going to get any better unless she starts to eat, which I seriously doubt because she said she can't."

"Well, I'll take ma chances. We can take care of her. I had to send my mama to a home, and you have no idea how that made me feel. I didn't have a choice then, but with my gal, I believe I do."

"For your sake, I hope you're right, Ms. Casey. I'll give her six weeks. If she makes it past those six, then she might make it."

Mama went back in the room where she was. Both of them looked as if they would cry at the snap of a finger, but they did not.

Mama said, "Well, you can go home."

"I might as well. There ain't nothin' he can do for me here."

Then the door opened. It was Dr. Jason again.

He said, "I changed my mind about letting you go home. I'm going to keep you in for another three days, and then you can go home."

Gent said, "You mean if I live that long."

He dropped his head and said, "Yes, if you live that long."

He put her on prednisone, USP, twenty milligrams. She had to take six a day. He told Gent that he knew he said that it couldn't be treated, but he was going to try anyway.

Mama called home to tell us the news. Essie was on her way up there before Mama got off the phone. She was talking to Aunt Kitty and told her that she wanted to speak to me before she hung up. I came to the phone. She spoke in a low, slow voice.

"Call Hubert and Ball. Tell 'em about Gent and see if they can come home."

"What's wrong? Why you sound like that? Ain't nothin' happen to Gent, did it?"

"I'll tell ya about it when I get there. I'm comin' home when Essie get here. She gon' stay wit Gent."

"All right, see ya later."

"Wait. Don't call 'em till I get home. I wanna tell 'em maself."

"Okay," I said, then hung up.

When Essie got to the hospital, Gent was just lying there. She wasn't saying anything. When Essie walked in, she didn't even look to see who it was. Mama and Essie went to the lobby so they could spend some time alone.

Essie asked Mama, "What was that you said she had?"

"Somethin' called lupus. Dr. Jason said that this is the first time he heard of it." She explained what it was to Essie.

"What he givin' her for it?"

"I don't know the name of the medicine, but she have to take six pills a day. He don't know if it'll do her any good. He ain't give her but six weeks to live. He said, if she make it them six weeks, that she might make it."

THE FIRST CASE OF LUPUS

Essie started pacing the floor and crying. She said over and over, "Lord, Lord, Lord. What we gon' do now. Don't take her away from us. Don't take her now."

Mama dropped her head but still held back the tears.

Meanwhile, back in the room, Gent was on the phone with Charlie, having their own little talk. She told him everything the doctor had told her and Mama. He felt so bad that he wasn't there with her.

He said, "Just hang in there, baby. I ain't got too much longer before I'll be back home. I wish I was there witcha."

"I wish you was too."

"You can make it. You got to. I can't lose you now."

They could hear each other crying on the phone. She had already hung up the phone before Mama and Essie came back in. They could tell that she had been crying. Neither of them said anything to her about it. Mama told her that she was getting ready to go and that she'd see her in the morning.

Before Mama left to go back to the hospital, Essie called home to see if she could change Mama's mind about staying another night. She told her that she needed to stay home and rest, but Mama said no and told her that she could stay the next night. So Essie agreed and hung up.

Mama came back with some clean clothes for Gent.

"You sure ya don't want me to stay tonight?" Essie said.

"Yeah. You can go on to the house."

"Okay. I'll see ya tomorrow, Gent."

"All right."

Mama said, "All the children asked about cha."

"I wanna see 'em so bad I don't know what to do."

"Well, ya know they all right."

"I know it, but I still wanna see 'em."

"You ain't got but a couple mo' days. Randy and Silver Jean wanna bring 'em 'round here to ya window for ya to see 'em."

"Tell 'em to bring 'em on. I'll sho be glad to see 'em."

"Did ya tell Charlie what the doctor said when ya talk to him?"

"Yeah. Whatcha'll talk about in the hall after ya left outta here?"

"Nothin' much. Just that I was gonna have to keep a close eye on ya when I getcha home. That's all."

"Well, whatever he told ya, tell Charlie 'cause he 'bout to worry his self to death."

"I know. All of us is. Tula was in the house when I was tellin' Kitty what the doctor said, and she bust out and started cryin'. When Charlie call back, I'll tell him."

"Tula ain't nothin' but a water barrel anyway."

They both gave a little laugh.

Mama told Gent that she had got in touch with Uncle Hubert and Ball and that they'd be home the following morning. They talked about where Gent would be sleeping.

She didn't want to sleep in the bed with Mama because she said it would be too crowded. Mama put her in the boys' room. They had to sleep in the front bedroom. She fixed it up for her on the day she didn't stay in the hospital.

After Mama helped Gent with her bath, she helped put on her gown, and Gent went right to sleep. Later in the night, Mama wanted something to drink. She figured that, since Gent was asleep, she could go to the snack room for a soda. While she was gone, Gent got out of bed and tried to go to the bathroom alone. She made it to the bathroom, but when she got ready to stand up, everything went black. She stood up, and the room started to spin. She lost her balance and fell. She hit her head on the bar in the bathroom and almost knocked herself out.

When Mama opened the door and saw that she wasn't in bed, she heard a noise in the bathroom. She ran over to the door and opened it. Gent was lying on the floor with a big knot shining on her forehead. Mama helped her get back to her bed.

"You know better than to try and go to the bathroom by yo'self. I was comin' right back, or either you coulda called for the nurse."

Gent said, "I know it, Mama. I just thought that I could do it by myself."

"What happened?"

THE FIRST CASE OF LUPUS

"I made it to the bathroom good. And after I used it, I got up to come back, and everything went black. I got dizzy and fell out. I could feel ma leg givin' out on me."

"The leg that they got that stuff out of?"

"Yes, ma'am."

"Do ya head hurt much?"

"No, ma'am. Not too much. Not till I try to move it off the pillow. Do it look bad?"

"Not too bad. But it ain't through swellin' yet. Don't try that no mo'. When I ain't here to help ya get up, you call the nurse. I ain't gonna leave ya alone no mo'."

Gent went back to sleep, and so did Mama after she made sure that Gent was. The next day, it was my turn to stay with her all day. Na took me and brought Mama back. Sterling wanted to know when he was gonna stay, but Mama told him that he couldn't because she needed somebody who could help her to the bathroom.

He said, "I can do that."

Mama said, "No. I'll get Randy to take you up there to see her tomorrow."

He walked off fussing.

When I got to her room and she turned around, I said, "What in the world happened to you?"

"I went in the bathroom and fell."

"How did it happen? You slipped?"

"No. I believe ma leg give out on me, then everything went black. I got dizzy, and that's all I remember till Mama came and got me off the floor."

"You gonna let the doctor know about it givin' out on ya?"

"I ain't gon' have to. He'll see this knot on ma for'ed."

"How long is it before you go home?"

"I suppose to go tomorrow or the next day."

"I know you ready to go. Do you want me to getcha anything?"

"Not right now, but I wantcha to go get me some cigarettes after a while."

"Okay."

"Mama said that Uncle Hubert was gettin' in this mornin'."

"He is. Ball supposed to be comin' wit him too."

"I wonder if he got in touch wit that crazy daddy of mine?"

"They mighta."

I got there way before visiting hours started, and when they did start, Aunt Kitty and Essie was the first to come. Essie was trying to talk me into letting her stay the day, but before I could say anything, Gent told her to let me stay and that she could stay that night and give Mama a break. She said okay and asked us if we had seen Hubert yet. We said no, and they stayed longer for a while talking to Gent and then left.

Gent had more visitors now than she ever had. Once word got out that the doctor only gave her six weeks to live, it was like everybody was coming to see her for the last time. People were in and out all that day.

It was eleven, and she told me that she was ready for me to go get her cigarettes. But first she wanted to go to the bathroom. I held her arm as she went. She couldn't pick her feet up. She had to slide them slowly. It took all the strength she had to do it. After she finished, I had to help her stand so that she could pull up her panties. Whenever she had a bowel movement, it was like fluid. That was because she never ate.

I helped her back into bed. She gave me the money, and I left.

When I got to the door, I turned to her and said, "Don't you try to get out of bed now."

She said, "Girl, don't cha worry. I learned my lesson."

As I was leaving the front entrance to the hospital, Uncle Hubert, Ball, and Gent's father were driving by. They saw me and stopped. They asked me where I was going. I told them.

All of them started telling me that she didn't need any and for me not to get them. I told them that I wouldn't, but I got them anyway. When I got back, they were in the room. I figured they had already talked to her about smoking, so I put the bag in the drawer. None of them were doing any talking. Gent was explaining to them what it was she had the best she could, and they only stood there and shook their heads. Her father's eyes were full of tears. All he had to do was blink. Ball let hers out. She had held it as long as she could.

THE FIRST CASE OF LUPUS

John D., her father, gave her $20 when they got ready to go.

Uncle Hubert looked at her and said, "If there's anything I can do for you, just let me know."

Then they left.

When he got to the door, he said, "She's a sick girl. Lord knows she is."

I walked them to the lobby.

When I got back to the room, Gent said, "Where ma cigarettes? Tellin' me I ain't got no business smokin'."

"They told me the same thing and told me not to getcha none."

"Shit. This $20 sho will come in handy. This is the first time he gave me money, and I didn't have to ask for it."

"They sho didn't do much talkin'."

"They ain't do none. Ya sister called from the lobby. She said that she would come back later, butcha know how that is."

She went to sleep after she did a few puzzles in the book I got for her. When she dozed off, I got the book and did one. I stopped and looked at her. All kinds of thoughts were running through my head. I felt like I was looking at a stranger. I didn't want to believe it was her, I guess. Everything about her had changed. She weighed only seventy pounds. She looked like an old lady who might have been in her eighties or nineties. She'd lost so much weight that I could almost tell where her joints were.

Her face was narrow and pointed. Her arms and legs were so skinny that her elbows were pointed and her kneecaps were the biggest part of her legs.

I left later that evening, and Aunt Essie came to spend the night. The next morning, Hubert, Ball, and John D. came back to see her. They were on their way back up north and wanted to see her before they left. They had more to say this time.

Hubert said, "Girl, I sho didn't know that you was this sick. If I had, I'da come home sooner."

"Me too, but Aunt Nank didn't call nobody and tell 'em nothin'," said Ball.

Her father looked at her and said, "How long have you been like this, and why didn't you let me know about it?"

She said, "I've been like this for about two or three months. It came on me slow at first."

Ball asked, "Are you in pain?"

She said, "No, not much. I ache in ma joints a little bit."

"Well, that's good. At least you're not in a lot of pain."

"Yep. When y'all leavin'?"

"We're on our way back now. We wanted to come by and see you again before we left," Hubert said.

"I hope to be goin' home maself tomorrow."

Hubert said, "Well, we're gonna go, so you can get some rest, okay?"

"Okay. Y'all have a safe trip."

He said, "We will, and you take care of yo'self and do what the doctor tell you to do. And another thing, try to stop smokin' please."

Gent smiled and said okay, but I knew she didn't mean it. As soon as they left, Mama came in. The first thing she asked was if the doctor had been in. Essie told her no, then she looked over at Gent and asked her how she was doing.

Gent always gave the same answer, "About the same."

Mama told Essie that she could go because she was there to stay with her.

Essie asked, "How you get up here?"

"Nathaniel brought me. He parked right out front," she said.

"All right, if ya want me to come back, just call to the house."

Mama said okay, and Essie left. At two thirty, the doctor came in. He checked her vital signs. Her fever was now very high. He told her to open her mouth. He took a little flashlight from his pocket and shined it in her mouth to see inside of it.

He said, "Geneva, I want you to try and drink at least a half a gallon of water a day. The fever has cooked your mouth on the inside, and I want you to drink the water so your mouth won't be so dry. Or maybe suck on some ice. I know it's going to be kind of hard to do, but you have to try."

He then went to the door and called for one of the nurses to bring a wheelchair.

THE FIRST CASE OF LUPUS

He looked at Gent and said, "I'm going to have them weigh you. After they do that, I don't see any reason why you can't go home. We just have to see what the meds will do for you."

Gent didn't want to go, but when he said something about going home, she didn't mind very much.

The nurse took Gent, and he stayed in the room and talked to Mama.

"Ms. Casey, have you thought about the talk we had the other day?"

"About what? Puttin' her in a home?"

"Yes, ma'am. That would be the best thing. She's going to have to have someone with her at all times. I don't know just how bad this disease can get her down or how much longer she may last. I'm releasing her because I don't think there's anything else we can do for her here."

"I gave ya ray answer then, and it's still the same."

"I don't know if the medication I'm giving her is helping any. It might be. Then again, it might not. I'm going to give her a prescription for it. I'm still keeping her on six a day. I'll be looking for you to bring her back any day after she leaves because this is new to me too. Good luck."

"Thank you."

When they got back to the room, Mama said, "How much did ya weigh?"

Gent gave her that you-won't-believe-it look but didn't say anything.

Dr. Jason looked at her records and said, "My Lord, sixty-six pounds!"

Mama's eyes got as big as a fifty-cent piece. She looked at Gent and shook her head. Gent still didn't say anything.

It was as hard for her to believe as it was for them.

Dr. Jason said, "Sixty-six pounds. A twenty-three-year-old woman weighing sixty-six pounds. Since you've been sick, you've lost a total of fifty-eight pounds. If you make it through this, Geneva, it'll be a miracle."

Mama said, "Yes, Lord."

"I'm going to the front desk and tell them to get your release forms together. I want you to try and eat something. I don't care what it is as long as you eat. Ms. Casey, give her what you can for the fever. I don't see how she's making it with it as high as it is. I hope that everything turns out okay for the sake of all of you."

Mama called Randy to pick them up. We were at the house fixing up the room they were going to sleep in. They had already moved in. Aunt Kitty and Na decided to rent the house that they had, and Cookie moved in with them.

After the move, Mrs. Deberry, the lady who owned the house Gent had been staying in, came home to see why she hadn't been getting any rent money. She came to the house, and Gent was sitting in the chair Mama had fixed for her.

She knocked on the door.

"Come in," Mama said.

She came in. "Hey, Nank, how ya doin'?"

"I'm fine, Mrs. Deberry. Come on in and have a seat."

"I wanted to see Gent. I went over to the house, but there won't anybody there," she said.

"There she is right there."

"No! How long she been like this?"

"Since April," said Mama.

Gent said, "It started before then, but it just got me this bad in April."

"Well, I'm sorry to hear that, but I would like to know what you gonna do about the rent money you owe me. You been stayin' in my house for more than eight months now, and I only got rent money from you three times."

"Well, there ain't no way I can pay it. I ain't been stayin' over there. I been here wit Mama since I been sick," Gent said.

"Well, I'll just have to take out a warrant because I need my money to pay my own bills."

Mama said, "I don't know whatcha gon' take it out on unless you take it out on the furniture 'cause she ain't been stayin' there."

"You said that she just moved out in April."

"She didn't. You can do whatcha wanna do, but she ain't goin' to jail."

"Well, I didn't come home to start no trouble. I just want ma money."

"I know ya didn't."

Then Aunt Kitty walked in. "Hi, how ya doin'?"

"I'm pretty good, Kitty. How you?"

"All right. I wanna talk to ya about somethin' when you get time."

Mama said, "Who?"

She said, "Mrs. Deberry."

"Oh, we can talk now if ya wanna."

"All right, let's walk out here."

When they left, Mama sat down in front of the fan with her sweat rag, wiping her face.

She said, "She better go sit her old ass down somewhere. She sound like a fool. I'll sue her and Dillon for puttin' you in jail, sick as you is. I'll beat her old ass."

Aunt Kitty asked her if she could rent the house since Gent wouldn't be staying in it.

"Yeah, 'cause I'ma tell Gent that she got to get her stuff out by the end of this week. Kitty, do you know that she ain't paid me for rent in almost six months?"

"I ain't surprised. She won't pay her bills now."

"Well, you can sho get it. I know you'll take care of it."

"All right, how much do I have to pay a month?"

"$50."

"Okay, let me pay for a month right now. I wanna get out on my own for a change."

"I know whatcha mean."

Mrs. Deberry left, and Aunt Kitty came back in the house to talk to Gent about the house.

She said, "Mrs. Deberry said that she told you to have yo' stuff out by the end of the week, so I decided to rent it. I didn't tell her that we had already started movin' in."

"Well, don't look like I'ma be stayin' there no mo' anyway."

"Is there anything there that you ain't gon' use?"

"I ain't got nowhere to put that stuff, but I'ma get ma TV and record player and put 'em in the room."

"I'ma take my bed in that back room. You can put one of yo' beds in the place of it."

"Okay."

"If ya don't need the rest of that stuff in there, I can use some of it."

"Okay. It's all right wit me."

On June 2, Charlie came home from basic training. He told Gent that he was only going to be home for three or four weeks. He had to go to Oklahoma for some kind of training, and he didn't know for how long. There wasn't too much that they could do for fun, but they made the best of the time they had.

It seemed like the weeks flew by. It was time for Charlie to leave before we knew it. Gent wanted to go with them to the bus station to see him leave. He and Randy put her in the car. When they got to the station, Charlie went to see what time the bus was coming, then went back to Gent.

"Well, babe, this is it. They said the bus should be here at any time now."

"You sure you got everything you need?"

"Yeah, I sho hate to leave you when you're feelin' so bad."

"Well, ya gotta go. Maybe time'll fly by like it did this time."

"I sho hope so."

Randy said, "Here she come."

"Yep," said Gent.

"I'll call and give ya number where I can be reached, okay?"

"Okay. I love you, and call me now."

"I will. Take care of yaself."

They kissed and said goodbye.

When they got back home, Gent told Randy to put on her record by Teddy Pendergrass. The name of it was "Close the Door." As soon as they got back, Tim came to see her.

She said, "Tim, Charlie gone now and won't be back again for four weeks."

THE FIRST CASE OF LUPUS

He said, "Is that a long time, Gent?"
"Yeah, baby. A whole month."
"Good. I told Ma you was my girlfriend anyway."
She laughed. "Whatcha mama doin' now?"
"She cookin'. You want some of what she cookin'?"
"No, Tim. I can't eat it."

He sat down on the floor next to her chair and was rocking his head to the music. Then he started rocking and trying to pop his finger, like he wanted to dance.

Then he said, "That's a bad record, ain't it, Gent?"
"Yeah, baby, it sho is."

After a while, we heard Cille calling him. "Tim, come home and eat. You can go back when you finish."

He got up to leave. "I'll be back, Gent," he said.

We didn't see him anymore that day.

Randy walked in and asked her how she was doing.

She said, "I'll do. I got a headache."

"You want a Goody's Powder?"

"Yeah, I sent over to Cille's for one, but she didn't have any."

He looked at me and said, "Silver Jean, take my car and go to the store and get her one. We'll get high when ya get back."

When I got back, Randy handed me the reefer and told me to roll three joints.

Gent said, "Randy, I wantcha to take me for a walk when you get time."

He said, "I better take ya after we finish this 'cause, if we wait, it'll be too hot."

"I'll walk as far as I can. You might have to tote me back."

"All right, no problem."

When we finished getting high, she and Randy went for their walk. Randy had her by the arm. She took each step slowly. She could pick her feet up a little better now than she could when she first came home. Mama was raking the yard when they left. She told Randy not to trust Gent too far alone because she didn't want her to fall.

She could walk as far as the front of her house, then Randy would have to pick her up and bring her back. He put her in the chair to rest, and Mama stopped raking to come in and talk to her.

"Mama, you ain't gotta stay in here wit me. Gwan back outside and finish the yards."

"No, child. Silver Jean or Sterling can finish them yards. I'ma sit in here and talk to you for a while."

"Where the children at?"

"Out there playing in the yard somewhere. When ya gon' talk to the woman aboutcha welfare check and them youngerns? You know ya ain't able to tend to 'em."

"I'ma call her in the morning and see if she'll come out here."

"Well, don't tell 'em thatcha already married. Tell her thatcha gettin' married."

"I am."

"She might wantcha to go up there and talk to her."

"No, she won't. All I got to do is tell her that I'm sick and ain't able to go up there, and she'll come out here."

Mama woke Gent up early the next morning to call her social worker. She helped her to the den where her chair was and gave her the phone. Gent looked at the clock, and it said eight.

She said, "I 'clare you mean for me to call her, don't cha?"

She said, "It's best to call her early so that she'll have time to come out here."

The phone rang six times before she got an answer. Finally, a voice came on the other end.

"Hello. Department of Social Services."

"Hi, this is Geneva Casey, and I'd like to speak to Terry Smith please."

"One minute please." She connected Gent with Terry's line.

She answered the phone.

"Hello, Terry speaking."

"Hi, this is Geneva Casey, and I'm calling to see if there's any way that you can come out here and see me today? I want to talk to you about turnin' my kids over to my mother."

"Why do you wanna do that, Geneva?"

THE FIRST CASE OF LUPUS

"I'm sick, and I'm not able to take care of them. I also wanted to talk to you about gettin' off of welfare because I'm gettin' married this week."

"Are you telling me that you want your mother to take your kids because you're sick and can't take care of them, but you're getting married this week?"

"Well, I can explain it better if you came out here and saw what I'm tryin' to tell you about."

"I think that would be best. I'll be out there in about two or three hours."

"All right, thank you," said Gent and hung up the phone.

Mama said, "What time is she comin'?"

"About eleven, when she take her lunch break."

"Let me go'n and cook so I'll be through when she get here. I'll probably have to sign some papers or somethin'."

"Ya might. Most likely you will."

At eleven thirty, Terry was pulling up in the yard.

Mama said, "Gent, she out there. You gon' stay in here, or is ya goin' on the porch?"

"It's kinda hot in here. Let's go on the porch."

"Okay, let me putcha a pillow in one of them chairs."

She put the pillow in the chair and came back to help her to it. While she was getting Gent ready, Terry was still in the car getting some papers together that she would need.

She got out the car and came on the porch. "I came to see Geneva. Is she here?"

Gent said, "Here I am."

Terry's mouth dropped open, and she turned as white as a ball of cotton. "Geneva, is that really you?"

"Yep, it's me."

"I didn't know who you were. How long have you been like this?"

"It's had me like this for about three or four months now. It started on me slow at first. I didn't think nothin' was wrong wit me until I lost so much weight and headaches wouldn't stop."

"Why haven't you gotten in touch with me before now?"

"Well, I've been in and out of the hospital this year, and I stayed on welfare to pay the bills and stuff."

"We could have arranged something. Your mother could have had the children, and you still could have been on welfare."

"I didn't know that."

"What did the doctor say was wrong with you?"

"I got a disease called lupus. It's a blood disease. They don't know what caused it, and there's no cure for it."

"My goodness! I hope you get better. Do they think you'll overcome it?"

"Well, they don't really know yet. He said that, if I could just eat something, it would help. But when they released me from the hospital, they said that they'd be lookin' for me to come back at any time."

"How long has it been since you've eaten anything?"

"About three or four months now."

"My God, how are you making it!"

"Wit the help of the good Lord."

"I'll just let you sign these papers, and you can go lie down. You'll have to sign some too, Ms. Casey."

"All right, just show me where," Mama said.

Terry couldn't take her eyes off of Gent. While Gent signed the papers, Terry watched her with a look of disbelief on her face. When they finished with the forms, they handed them back to her.

She took them and said again, "I hope you get better, Geneva. Take care of yourself now. Goodbye." She got in her car and left.

When she got to the office, she called back to the house. Mama answered the phone.

"Hi, this is Terry. I meant to tell you while I was out there that this month's check will be in Geneva's name. It's too far in the month to have it put in your name."

"All right."

"Okay, Ms. Casey. Bye now."

Gent had me put on her Teddy Pendergrass's album.

Mama said, "Oh, Lord, there it goes again."

Gent said, "If you don't wanna hear it, Silver Jean can turn it off."

THE FIRST CASE OF LUPUS

"No, honey, I was just kiddin'. You can play yo' music all you want to. It ain't botherin' me."

"I have to listen to ma man sing. That's what keeps me going now that Charlie ain't here."

She had a picture of him that she kept with her all the time.

While her record "Close the Door" played, she looked at the picture and said, "Lord, that's a sweet man there."

Mama said, "You love that ole long, tall nigger, don't you?"

"Yeah. That's my baby. I miss him too."

"I know ya do."

After Charlie left, Gent got worse. Her hair came out more, and she lost more weight. Her nerves started messing up on her too. When she would get ready to return a letter to Charlie, she'd have me write it for her. Her nerves had her shaking so bad she couldn't even write her name.

When Charlie got her letter, he called home. He wanted to know how she was doing. The day he called, Mama answered the phone.

"Hello."

"Collect call from Luther Taylor. Will you accept?" the operator asked.

Mama said, "Hold on a minute." She turned to Gent and said, "Who is Luther Taylor?"

Gent laughed and said, "Mama, that's Charlie."

Mama said, "Child, I didn't know." Then she put the phone back to her ear and said, "Yes, I will."

Charlie said, "Hey, how ya doin'?"

"Pretty good, and you?"

"I'll make it, I reckon. Where's Gent at?"

"Right here. Let me give her the phone." She handed her the phone.

Gent said, "Hey."

"Hey, sweets, how ya doin'?"

"I'll make it. How 'bout you?"

"Why ya voice sound like that?"

"I believe ma nerves tryin' to mess up on me. It ain't nothin' too serious, I hope."

"You better have yo'self checked to see if it is gonna do any harm. I'll be home in three or four weeks, and I want you to be doin' a little better than you was when I came here."

"Well, I ain't gonna promise ya that I am."

"Ya better gawn and have ya butt checked. You ain't to worry 'bout no bills. You know that."

"Yeah, I know it. I might go. It's a little better than it was."

"Oh, you just don't wanna go."

"Well, you know they can't do nothin' for me, so what's the use in goin'?"

"I don't know."

"How do you like it out there?"

"It's all right. I met a few people I know. I met this dude from Latta."

"Well, it shouldn't be too bad."

"It ain't. I'm just homesick mostly. How is everybody doin'?"

"All right."

"Sterling still 'round there gittin' high?"

"Every chance he get."

"Well, I just called to see how you were doin'. I'ma go now, but I'ma write in a couple of days and send ya some money. Then you can pay Mama for this call, okay?"

"All right, I'll be lookin' for ya letter. Bye."

"Bye, and take care of yo'self. Love ya."

Mama came in and said, "What he wanted? To see how you was doin'?"

"Yes, ma'am. I guess he got worried when he saw that the letter I sent won't in my handwritin'."

"I reckon he is worried about his wife."

"I'll sho be glad when he come home. I'm gittin' tired of lookin' at a picture. It can't talk back."

Mama laughed and said, "The way you look at it, you act like it talk back."

"Well, it's the next best thing besides that phone call I just got."

THE FIRST CASE OF LUPUS

"How he like it out there?"

"He said it was okay. He gonna send me some money next week so I can pay you for that call."

"I ain't worried about that call, but them few dollars sho will come in handy. I know he gon' call and check on ya, so I look for that."

I started her record over for her, and Mama got up to go and rake yards.

She asked Mama, "Where you goin'?"

"Out here in the yard. Why? You want somethin'?"

"No. I just wanted to know where you was goin'," she said in a shaky voice.

Gent was worse than a small child. Whenever Mama would get somewhere in the yard where Gent couldn't see her, she would call her and say, "Mama, where you at?"

Mama would say, "Right here."

She'd say, "Where? I can't see ya."

Then Mama would walk back over in front of the door where she could see her and say, "Here. I'm right here."

She'd start raking there in front of the door, and as soon as she was out of Gent's eyesight, she'd hear her call her again.

I was sitting on the porch, and Mama looked at me and said, "Lord, I can't rake yards till she go to sleep."

"I'll rake 'em this evenin' when it cool off some," I said.

She put the rake down and went in the house.

Gent said, "Ya musta got hot out there?"

"Yeah, it's hotter than I thought it was."

"When do Aunt Kitty them start puttin' in 'bacco?"

"I believe George said they was gon' start next week."

I yelled from the porch, "I'll sho be glad."

"I wish I was able to put in some," Gent said.

Mama said, "Well, you know you can't, so don't worry about it."

Charlie called back again that night. He told Gent that he was going to send some papers, along with the money, she would have to fill out and send back to him. When she got the papers, she found out that she had to get her birth certificate and she had to go to Fort Bragg and get an ID card made.

Mama went the next day and got her birth certificate for her. When Mama got back, we found out that her name was Jeanette Joyce Casey instead of Geneva Joyce.

She looked at Mama and said, "Mama, you mean to say that you didn't even know what ma name was?"

Mama laughed and said, "Child, I knew it was somethin' like that. I ain't gonna lie. I thought it was Geneva too."

"I know Charlie gon' trip offa this. He gon' swear that I didn't know ma own name."

"Hell, ya didn't."

All of us laughed. When she told Cille about it, she did give her a fit.

She said, "You better not send that thang to that man without explainin' it to him first. He'll swear out that he don't know ya."

Gent and Mama laughed, thinking about how he would react when he got it.

That night, Mama called Uncle Thomas and told him that they had to take Gent to Fort Bragg to have her ID card made. He said for her to come to the house and he would take them straight to the place.

We got up early the next morning and left. Gent lay down most of the way there. When we got there, Randy helped her into the house. Uncle Thomas had made some spaghetti and told us to sit down and eat because the place she had to go to wasn't open yet. Aunt Clovis told Gent to go in her room and lie across the bed, but she said no because she was lying down all the way up there.

At eight fifty, Uncle Thomas said that he was ready.

He said, "By the time we get there, the place should be open. Hope for your sake we'll be the first one there and can go on in."

Randy said, "I'll wait here till ya get back."

"Don't cha drank too much where ya won't be able to drive back home. I ain't drivin'," Mama said and walked out the door.

THE FIRST CASE OF LUPUS

When we got there, there was only a couple of people there. Mama bought a pillow just in case the chairs didn't have cushions in them. We sat on the first row of seats.

Uncle Thomas put the papers on the desk and signed her name on the list.

He came back to sit down and said, "It shouldn't be too long. She's the fourth one on the list."

Mama said, "Good. After sittin' down too long, her butt'll start hurtin'."

We sat there for twenty or thirty minutes, and then they called her.

"Jeanette Taylor."

Mama went to her and grabbed her by the arm.

The man that was waiting on her asked, "Do you need some help, ma'am?"

"No, thank you. I got her."

She went in the office and sat down.

He said, "Mrs. Taylor, why did you come with you being as sick as you are?"

"My husband told me to get the papers back as soon as I could, so I came on up here to get it over with."

"Well, we'd better go on and get started so you can go home and rest, but you could've sent us a picture, and we could have made the card from that."

"I didn't know that. I thought that maybe I had to sign some papers or somethin'."

"No, you could have explained your situation and sent in a picture. We usually have them stand to have their picture made, but I'm going to let you sit. Here's your chair."

She sat down. He took the picture and told her to go back to the waiting room and the person at the desk would call her for her card. We only had to wait about five minutes, then they called her. I went and got the card. Mama and Uncle Thomas were helping Gent out the door.

When we got to the car, Mama said, "Let me see how the picture turned out."

Gent said, "No, ya don't." She snatched it from me. "I ain't lettin' nobody see this ugly thang."

"Well, the camera took what it saw," said Mama.

"That's why nobody ain't seein' it. They can look at me."

When we got to the house, Randy and Aunt Clovis asked her if they could see it. She told them no too. On the way home, she handed it to Mama. Mama didn't say anything. She just started laughing.

Gent said, "I knew you was gonna laugh."

Mama said, laughing, "Lord, it ain't nothin' to laugh about, but you look like a big 'bacco worm."

She didn't look anything like herself on the card. She didn't want to send it to Charlie either, but she knew that she had to.

Mama picked at her about that card for a week. Whenever anybody would come to the house, Mama would tell them to ask Gent to let them see the picture.

Gent would just say, "I ain't thinkin' 'bout you. Let them see yo' picture."

Mama would start laughing. I think she was laughing to keep from crying.

Mama would say, "Tell Charlie to put it in the back of his wallet and don't show it to nobody."

Like always, Gent didn't pay any attention to her.

The next week came, and we started to work. Every morning when we got up, Gent would already be awake. When she had money to spare, she made sure that she gave Ma and Sterling enough to get us something with. Sterling was always the first one to ask 'cause she was more like a mother to him instead of a sister.

He didn't sit around her as much as I did or Randy.

He didn't like seeing her like that. On days when we didn't have to work, he'd be out somewhere playing ball. He'd go look in on her every day though. He wouldn't stay long, just long enough to see how she was doing.

She loved macaroni and cheese, and every day after work, I'd go in her room and ask her if she was ready for me to make her some. She'd say no and that she'd rather wait till the next night.

THE FIRST CASE OF LUPUS

We were about halfway finished putting in tobacco that year. It was on a Wednesday, and we had just started back for that evening. We were putting in Mr. Jack's tobacco.

His son came to the barn at about three and said, "One of Bopete's sons just drowned."

Bopete was Cille's husband.

Aunt Kitty said, "Which one?"

"They said it was the one 'bout eight or nine."

I said, "That would be Marvin 'cause Tim ain't but five and Darren is eleven."

"They said it was the baby boy."

"Oh, God. Well, it must be Tim," I said.

"Where did it happen at?" asked Aunt Kitty.

"Right there in front of that field's girl's house."

"Must be that irrigation pond next to Clay's house. God, I hate that. I know Cille's about to have a fit," I said.

"Ya know she is," said Aunt Kitty.

"I wonder if anybody told Gent?"

"I doubt if Nank told her."

Tootsie said, "Well, I'ma go. I just come to tell y'all the news."

We all said all right, and he left. Tim's death was the talk for the rest of that day. When we got home from work, the wreath was already on the door. There were a few people standing out in the yard when we drove up.

When we got home, Mama had all of the curtains pulled together. Gent had been back in Mama's room lying down, but as soon as we got home, she wanted to get up and sit in her chair for a while. When we got her in her chair, I went over to open the curtains. Mama called me and shook her head no, telling me not to open them.

Gent said, "God, whatcha got the curtains closed for, Mama? Ya can't see nothin' sittin' in here."

Mama said, "As hot as it is out there, I thought that, if I'd close the curtains, it would feel a little cooler in here."

"It cools off anyway this time of the day. Shoot, I be wantin' to see the outside sometime."

So Mama said, "Go'n and open 'em, Silver Jean."

Aunt Kitty went to Mama and told her that Gent couldn't see over to Cille's house anyway with the curtain open. She also said somebody should be on the porch to tell the people who come to see Gent not to say anything about Tim. Mama went and sat out there herself since Essie was in the house with Gent. Essie wanted to tell her, but Mama told her not to.

I was in my room taking a bath. I got dressed to go to the settin' up for a while.

When I came out, Gent said, "What you all dressed up for? You ain't goin' out tonight, is ya?"

I said, "No, Bobby Gene comin', and we goin' to the Pizza Hut."

"Bring me a piece back."

"For what? You ain't gon' eat it."

"Just bring it back. You'll see."

I went to the settin' up. I didn't stay very long. When I got back, Gent was back in Mama's room in the bed. She called me 'round there and asked where her pizza was.

"We changed our mind. We didn't go to the Pizza Hut. We went to Weiner King instead," I said.

"Well, ya still coulda brought me somethin' back. Where Cookie at?"

"In the yard or home, one," I said.

"Tell her to send me a cigarette."

I told her, and she went into the house to get it. I went into the room where Gent was, and then she called Bobby in there too. When Cookie came in, we sat in there and acted like fools with Gent for a long time.

Then she said, "I want that macaroni and cheese that you supposed to be makin' for me now, Silver Jean."

I said, "I'ma make it, and you better eat it too."

"I am. Soon as it get done, bring me some in a plate."

Bobby said, "And if ya don't eat it, I'ma help her feed it to ya."

Gent laughed. They stayed in the room and talked while I made the macaroni. When I finished, I put some on a plate and took it to her. She ate two spoonfuls and told me to put the rest in the oven.

THE FIRST CASE OF LUPUS

The next morning, after we went to work, Mama told her about Tim. She went into her room and sat on the bed next to her.

She rubbed her face gently and said, "Gent, I got some bad news for ya. Now I don't wantcha to get upset."

"What is it?" she asked.

"Try not to get upset 'cause it won't help ya none."

Gent's eyes widened, and she said, "Ain't nothin' happen to none of the children, did it?"

"No. Tim drowned yesterday in that pond by Clay's house."

Gent started screaming and shaking her head. "No, Mama!"

She sat up and then started to get up. Mama tried to hold her back, but she pushed her aside and got up and went for the front door. When she got to it, she started to fall. Johnny, Essie's boyfriend, caught her.

She said to him, crying, "Help me to the door."

He grabbed her by the arm and helped her to it. When she got there, she looked over at Cille's and saw the wreath on the door. She fell back on Johnny and cried even harder. She kept saying over and over that she couldn't believe it. Mama told Johnny to bring her back and put her in the bed, He picked her up and put her back in bed.

Essie lay next to her, trying to calm her down. "Hush and stop that cryin'. Thank the Lord for not takin' you."

She said, crying, "Lord, that po' baby gone. It coulda been me. Look at how sick I am. He was just a baby."

"Well, hush now. It was just his time. The Lord know what He doin'."

Mama went over to see how Cille was doing, and while she was there, she told her that she had told Gent about Tim.

Cille asked, "How did she take it?"

"Not good. She been cryin' and goin' on ever since I told her."

"Let me go see this girl. I don't want nothin' to happen to her."

She and Mama came back to the house. When Gent saw her, she started to cry even more. Cille asked her how she was doing. Gent asked her the same thing.

"I'm fine. I came to make sure you were all right," said Cille.

"You didn't have to do that. You got problems of ya own."

"Yeah, but mine was done by the Lord. Yours was done by you gettin' all upset."

"I can't help it. That was ma baby," said Gent.

"I know it."

Mama said, "If there's anything I can do for ya, Cille, let me know."

"That goes for any of us," said Essie.

"Thank y'all, but I think we got everything 'bout straightened out."

When we got home for dinner, Cille was just leaving.

We went into the room where Gent was, and she was still crying. I and Cookie didn't stay. We went over to Cille's house to see how she was doing. We talked about Gent and how we thought she might handle the news. We stayed longer for a while and left. When we left to go back to work, Gent had stopped crying, and she was just lying there without saying anything.

We got through that day early. About three, Gent was sitting in her chair. We couldn't hardly understand a word she said. It was like she had to force her words out.

She said, "I…want…you…and…Cookie…to…take…me…to…the…sittin' up…tonight."

I said, "God, you can hardly getcha words out."

"You ain't kiddin'," said Cookie.

Aunt Kitty said, "Ya nerves messed up on ya again?"

"Yes…ma'am. I got…too…upset."

"Well, Nank wanted to tell ya instead of ya hearin' it from somebody else."

"That…thang…sho…hurt…me. I…couldn't…believe…it."

"Well, don't try to talk."

"The funeral is Sunday, and I'ma try to be there," said Cookie.

I said, "I doubt if I'm goin'."

"Me either," said Mama.

Gent wasn't able to go to the funeral. She was willing to try, but Mama wouldn't let her. Aunt Kitty, Essie, Cookie, and all the kids except Ficky went. Gent cried as if she were there though. Mama

THE FIRST CASE OF LUPUS

kept telling her to stop crying so much 'cause she wasn't doing anything but making herself worse.

"Mama, I can't help it. I still can't believe he's gone. He came to see me every day," Gent said.

"Yeah, he gone, but you gotta take care of yo'self now. The good Lord takin' care of him."

"I know it, but it still hurts."

"Well, ya gotta calm down. That's all there is to it."

When they got back from the funeral, Gent had already calmed down and was watching TV. Cookie handed her the obituary. As she read it, she began to cry again.

Cookie said, "Dog, girl, if I knew you was gonna start cryin', I wouldn't have gave it to ya."

She said, "Girl...that...was...ma...baby. I...can't...help...it."

"Yeah, it got the best of me too."

"Was the funeral sad much?" asked Mama.

"Yes, ma'am. Darren and Marvin took it real hard. Well, all of 'em took it hard. Cille would've killed ya."

Aunt Kitty said, "Yes, Lord. I couldn't hardly stand it."

"I hate...I...won't...there...for ma...buddy," Gent said.

"She understand thatcha won't able to go," Aunt Kitty said.

Cookie said, "All three of the boys was dressed just alike."

Mama said, "Lord have mercy. It's somethin' to lose somebody thatcha brought into this world."

I came in the room. "Bopete cut his hair."

"He did?" asked Aunt Kitty.

Is that where he had you to take him the other day when he asked you to drive for him?" asked Mama.

"No, ma'am. He went and got the boys' suits. He didn't cut his hair till the day before they put him out. He said that he didn't want nobody else to do it."

"Ain't that sweet. I don't believe I coulda did it," said Mama.

"Lord, that Tula know she did some cryin' today," said Aunt Kitty.

"I...know...she...did.   The...least...little...thing...that...hurt...her...feelins', she...start...cryin'. Where...Essie...at? Still...

at…the… church…tryin'…to…calm…every…body…down?" asked Gent.

"She stayed to go to the grave. We caught a ride back with Jill."

The day after the funeral, Cille came over to see Gent. She was sitting in the den and saw her when she came up on the porch.

When she knocked on the door, Gent said, "Come…on…in…Cille."

She came in. "Hey, how ya doin' today?"

"Pretty…good. I…should…be…askin'…you…that."

"Well, I'm makin' it, by the help of the Lord."

"Girl…I…sho…hate…that…'bout…ma…baby."

"Yeah. Why you talkin' like that?"

"Ma…nerves…goin'…bad…on…me. They…had…started…messin'…up…on…me…one…time…befo, but…when…I…heard…'bout…Tim, it…got…worse."

"You better take care of yo'self. I don't want nothin' to happen to you. I couldn't stand another funeral. Not right now."

"All right…Cille. Don't…talk…like…that."

"You know, Gent, I believe Tim saw death."

"What…cha…mean?"

"Ya know for yo'self that, when Bopete tell them boys not to leave out the yard, they won't leave."

Mama came in to see what she was talking about.

"Well, he told Tim not to, and he had already told him one time before. And as soon as Bopete went back in the house, Tim left again."

"Yeah…they…listen…to…him…now…'cause…they…know…he'll… cut…they…butt," said Gent.

"And you know that hot cycle I bought him for his birthday? He said that he didn't need it and for me to give it to Madie or Toot-Toot. I didn't pay him any attention. And later on that same day, me and him was sittin' on the porch talkin', and he said, 'Ma, I saw where Gent goin'. She goin' to a pretty place.' And I still didn't pay him any attention. You know how children always talkin' fool talk. That's all I thought it was."

THE FIRST CASE OF LUPUS

Mama said, "Lord, that baby saw heaven. He said that Gent was goin' there, but he saw his own death and didn't know it."

Cille looked like she wanted to cry. Then she said, "Bopete beat him 'bout goin' to Clay's house, but he went back anyway. Clay said that she told him to go back home before he got a beatin', and he said that he won't gettin' no beatin' 'cause Bopete knew that he was down there. At about two, Munk came to the house and said that Tim was in the irrigation hole. Girl, I couldn't move. I told Bopete to go see what he was talkin' about 'cause my baby won't in that hole."

"Did Bopete see him when he went down there?" asked Mama.

"No, not till the rescue squad got down there and pulled him out. They said that they had to get him out of a hole."

"What…in…the…world…was…he…doin'…in…there?" asked Gent.

"I don't know. Them children said that he went in after his ball. Ralph said he tried to pull him out, but his hand slipped out of his. And when Tim went down that time, he didn't come up no mo'."

Mama said, "I don't know what them ole people put that hole 'round here for anyway wit all these children 'round here."

"I don't either, Nank," said Cille.

"But that baby felt death. There won't no way he could shake it. If it's meant for ya, ya can't run from it."

"Yeah, Nank, ya right about that. Bopete was there when they pulled him out. He identified the body. I just couldn't go down there. When he came back to the house, he stood in the yard and cried like a baby. I knew right then that Tim was gone."

Mama got up and went back into the kitchen with tears rolling down her face. I looked over at Tula, and she was crying too. Gent wiped a few tears from her eyes.

Cille said, "Let me go. I didn't mean to come over here and get y'all started."

"I…can't…help…but…think…about…it. That…coulda… been…me. Just…look…at…how…sick…I…am…and…won't… nothin'…wrong… wit…him."

"My ma always said, 'Sickness don't mean death,'" said Mama.

Gent and Cille both agreed.

"Well, I'ma go," Cille said. "I feel a little better since I talked about it."

"Sometimes it helps to talk about things like that," said Mama.

"It sho do. Well, I'ma see y'all tomorrow. If I ain't back befo' then."

Gent said, "All right…I'm…glad…ya…came…by. Take…care…of…yaself…now."

Time passed; and for Gent, things weren't getting any better, not yet anyway. To make things worse, Mama wasn't resting very much either. She told Aunt Kitty that she'd lie in bed at night sometimes listening to Gent breathe.

She said that she sounded like every breath was going to be her last one. Aunt Kitty told her that she shouldn't do that because she was going to end up making herself sick.

"I can't help it. That's my child," Mama said.

It was now the end of July. Mama was in the kitchen cooking, and Gent and Randy were in the room where she slept, listening to Teddy Pendergrass.

Mama asked Gent, "If I make you a cake, will ya eat some of it?"

She said, "I'll do ma best to try. What kind ya makin'? Chocolate?"

"Yeah. That's the kind ya want, dontcha?"

"Yes, ma'am."

Randy said, "Well, I would stay in here and talk a little while longer, but I'm 'bout to go to sleep. I'll see ya when I wake up. I ain't gon' sleep too long 'cause I wanna get some of that cake befo' it get gone."

"All right, man," she said.

He left and went to bed.

Aunt Essie went in to talk to her. "You feelin' any better today, or 'bout the same?"

"Feel like I got worse."

"Well, just lie there and rest then."

It was about eleven thirty in the morning, and she stayed in her room alone after Randy and Essie left. We thought she was asleep, so we left her alone to rest. Mama was mixing the cake while standing in

THE FIRST CASE OF LUPUS

front of the door to the room Gent was in when she heard Gent. She was gasping for air, and her hands were stretched out, reaching for the ceiling. Mama looked and hollered her name. By the time Mama got to her, she had turned on her side.

Mama started shaking her and calling her name. Her eyes were rolled back in her head, and she was foaming at the mouth. All of us ran into the room to see what was wrong.

Mama stopped shaking her and ran out the room, crying, "Lord, she gone. My baby gone!"

One of Aunt Essie's old boyfriends had come by to see her. They were in the living room talking. When Mama started hollering, they came out asking what was wrong.

Randy jumped out of bed and came in with his pants halfway on and followed Essie and Mr. Townsend into Gent's room.

She had stopped breathing.

Essie went outside hollering and crying and looking for Mama; but Mama had run down the road, still crying, "My baby gone."

Mr. Townsend said, "Randy, blow in her mouth and try to get some air in her lungs while I pump her chest."

Na called the rescue squad. Randy breathed a few times and stopped to see if she was breathing yet, and she wasn't.

Mr. Townsend said, "Don't stop. Try it again."

He kept on pumping. Finally, her eyes returned to their normal position, and she took her hand and pushed Randy's head away. Then we heard the ambulance pull up.

She looked as if she was in another world.

Randy was rubbing her face, saying, "Can ya hear me, Gent? You all right?"

Aunt Kitty was crying and trying to get the kids calmed down. Mama came back when she saw the ambulance, but she didn't come into the house. I tried to calm her down by telling her that she was all right, but it didn't do any good. I tried to hug her and tell her to stop crying, but she only pushed me away.

When the ambulance came, people came from everywhere. Most of the people there were crying. Nobody thought they were going to see Gent alive again.

Na asked, "Who gonna go wit her in the rescue squad?"

I said, "I'll go."

Cookie said, "I'ma go too."

They put her on the stretcher and rolled her out the door. Everybody tried to get a quick look at her before she left. Na got in his car to follow us to the hospital. Aunt Essie went to the other door to open it and get in, but he locked it.

She said, "Lord, nobody won't take me to my Gent."

Na said, "They don't need nobody up there hollerin' and cuttin' the fool."

Aunt Kitty said, "The first thing you hear, call and let us know."

All the way to the hospital, we didn't say anything. Gent stared at us like we were strangers. I wanted to touch her, but I didn't know how she would react.

We were in the hospital before Na was because he had to find a parking space. When he came in, he was crying.

He said, "Where they take her at? Back there?"

We said, "Yeah."

He went back to her room. She was lying there with her eyes open but wasn't responding to anyone.

Na put her hand in his and said, "Ya gotta try and eat. Ya just gotta. Ya children need ya. We need ya. Don't give up, Gent. Please don't." He put his head down on the bed beside her and cried.

Then he heard her say, "What happen? Where I'm at?"

He began to cry harder and said, "I thought we was gonna lose ya one time. Ya had all of us worried."

"Who up here witcha?"

"Silver Jean and Cookie."

"Tell Head to come here."

He came and told me that she wanted me.

I said, "She do! Come on, Cookie. Both of us can go."

When we went in, she was looking up at the ceiling.

She said, "Y'all found ya hearts yet?"

Cookie said, "Girl, I believe I left mine in Riverdale."

I said, "I believe mine just gettin' back together. Girl, I was scared to death."

THE FIRST CASE OF LUPUS

"I know Mama like to had a fit," she said.

"Girl, everybody was cryin'. It was a time back in that hole," said Cookie.

"Mama said that you was dead. If it won't for Mr. Townsend and Randy, you mighta been," I said.

"Maybe now I'll live a long life since I already been pronounced dead. I'ma do ma best to anyway."

"I hope the Lord ya do," I said.

"I don't remember nothin' that happened. The last thing I remember was Randy tellin' me that he was goin' to bed. And that's all."

"I don't see how Mama heard you because she had the mixer on. Essie had the record player on in the living room."

"There was a lot of noise in the house 'cause the children was in there playin' too" Cookie said.

"Nank can hear now. I want some chicken, so I wantcha to call her, Head, and tell her to bring ma pocketbook. It's under my pillow."

"Okay, I'll be right back."

I got a dime from Na to call. Aunt Kitty answered the phone.

When she said hello, I could hear Mama in the background saying, "Don't tell me. If she gone, don't tell me. I don't wanna hear it. Just don't tell me."

I said, "Tell Mama Gent's all right. She told me to tell Mama to bring her, her pocketbook. It's under her pillow on her bed. She said that she wanted some chicken."

When Aunt Kitty told her what I said, I could hear her and Essie hollering, "Thank you, Jesus. You gave her to me for a while longer."

Mama couldn't drive, so she got a friend of the family, Mr. Dale, to bring her. On her way up there, she told him to stop by the liquor store so she could get something to calm her nerves. Beep picked at her because she didn't drink. She told him that this was something to drink for. They both agreed with her.

By the time Mama got to the hospital, Na had already talked to the doctor, and they had put Gent in her room. She gave Na the money for the chicken, and he went to the Colonel and got it. When he got back with it, we didn't leave. We stayed to see if she was really going to eat it, and she did—every piece of it.

Essie met us at the door when we got back. She asked, "How she doin'?"

Na said, "I think she gonna make it."

"What did the doctor say?" asked Aunt Kitty.

Na just shook his head and walked off.

Aunt Kitty said to the kids, "Ya mama gonna be all right."

"She ate a box of chicken before we left," I said.

Cookie said, "She was cuttin' wit that thang."

Aunt Kitty was so happy to hear that she started crying again. The whole time all that was going on with Gent, Sterling was sitting on the patio. He didn't even move when they put her in the ambulance. He just sat there and watched. When he heard that she was all right, he was too.

They didn't keep her in the hospital long. He told her to just keep on taking her medicine as prescribed.

In a couple of days, she was back home. Slowly but surely, she began to gain a few pounds. Her fever went away, and each day, she ate a little more. She ate more cereal than anything.

It had been a long time since she smoked any dope, and Mama didn't want her to. Randy went into her room one day and asked her if she wanted to try some.

She said, "Yeah, but I can't let Mama see me."

"Tell her thatcha gotta go to the bathroom, and I'll help ya."

Randy went back in the den, and Gent told Mama what Randy had told her to.

Mama said, "All right, I'm comin'."

Randy jumped up and said, "I'll help her."

He helped her to the bathroom and put down the toilet lid, and she sat down on it. He handed her the joint, and she lit it. She couldn't hold in the first pull. Na was sitting in the den, and he heard her coughing. He started laughing. The next pull was the same way. They smoked only one. When they came out, she told him to sit her

THE FIRST CASE OF LUPUS

in her chair. Before she got to it, she leaned up against the bar and shook her head.

Randy said, "That's some good shit, ain't it?"

"You ain't wrong. Maybe it hit me so hard 'cause I ain't had none in a while."

"Yeah, that might be it, but it is good."

Na said, "I swear ya can't keep the bummer down."

"Oh no," said Randy.

Fifteen minutes later, Gent said she wanted some cornflakes. We didn't have any at the house.

Mama said, "Let me get my gal her cornflakes. I'm so glad to see her eatin' I don't know what to do. Here, Randy, go to the store and get 'em."

"Mama, I swear I don't wanna go to the store. Not right now anyway."

"Well, give Silver Jean the keys then. Somebody gonna go 'cause the doctor said, whenever she want somethin' to eat, to try and get it for her."

I got the keys and left. When I got back, Gent told me to fix her some. Mama told me not to give her but a cupful because she might not eat it all. When I handed her the cup, she looked at me like I was crazy.

She said, "What's that?"

I said, "Yo' cornflakes."

"No, it ain't either. Not that little bit. You musta thought I wanted them for Ricky?"

Randy fell over on the chair laughing.

"Mama told me not to give ya too much 'cause ya might not eat 'em."

"I want a bowl. The yellow one in the cabinet."

I went back to get the bowl and gave it to her.

"Now that's more like it."

Randy looked at her, laughing, and said, "Ya got the munches, ain't cha?"

She said, "Yeah, boy."

Mama came in and looked at Na. She started laughing when she looked at Gent, then she turned to Na and said, "She cuttin', ain't she?"

"You ain't kiddin'," he said.

Aunt Essie went back home, taking most of Gent's wedding presents with her. She said that she was making sure no one was going to mess with them.

Charlie called to see how she was doing and to let her know how things were going with him. She told him about the incident that sent her to the hospital. He was glad that he wasn't here at the time but wanted to know about how the family was coping.

He asked, "Is Essie still down there?"

"No. She left last week. She wanted me to stay a week wit her, but there ain't no way I was gonna stay in Bladenboro a whole week."

"I know whatcha mean."

"Where did they station you at?"

"I don't know yet. I'll be home for three weeks, and then I gotta go to Fort Stewart in Georgia and sign some papers. I might be stationed down there."

"It sho would be nice if ya could get at Fort Bragg. That way, we won't be so far away from home."

"I tried, but I couldn't. Georgia was ma second choice."

"Well, I guess that ain't too bad. Georgia ain't but, what, a three- or four-hour drive?"

"Somethin' like that."

They enjoyed the three weeks Charlie had home, and time seemed to fly. Before we knew it, it was time for him to go. Before he left, he told Gent that, the next time he came home, they would be going back together.

She didn't say anything until after he left.

She looked at Mama and said, "He don't know if I'm goin' or not. That's too far from home."

Mama laughed. "You know you ain't goin' nowhere till you get better. Charlie just pickin' atcha. And when ya go, you ain't gon' go by yo'self."

"Who gon' go wit me?"

"Who ya want to go witcha?"

"Well, I want Head to go, but she gotta go to school. I'll probably take Ricky wit me, but I don't know yet."

A few days later, Charlie called and told her that he would be stationed in Georgia permanently. She told him not to be in a hurry to find anywhere to stay because she didn't want to try to make it at home alone until she got better. He said he knew that already.

As the days passed, Gent got better. The better she got, the faster the days seemed to pass. In three months, Gent had eaten way back to 125 pounds.

The first week in November, Charlie called and said that he was coming home. From what he read in her letters, Gent was ready and able to make Georgia her home, but he didn't tell her that until he got home.

When he walked in the door, he hugged her and gave her a kiss and said, "Ya ready to go to ya new home?"

She said, "Whatcha mean?"

"I found us a trailer. The rent is $125 a month. All we got to do is move in."

"You mean go back when you go Sunday?"

"Yep. Is that a problem?"

"I got to get ma final checkup Tuesday mornin'. I can go next week," she said.

She didn't really have to get a checkup. She just wasn't ready to go yet.

He said okay and that he'd be back the following week to get her. They talked about where they'd be living. Gent had all kind of questions to ask him, but there was one that she wanted a definite answer to.

"Can I come home at least twice a month?"

He said that they could.

The week passed quickly. Before we knew it, Charlie was back home helping Gent pack up her things to move. It was her last weekend at home, and she stayed high every chance she got. On the day they left, she cried like a baby, and so did Mama. All of us hated to see her go. Sterling went outside around the house to do his crying.

He wanted to go with her, but Mama told him that he had to go to school.

Ricky didn't want to go, but she took him anyway. He started crying. Mama told them to go on. He would quiet down farther down the road. Von got mad because Ricky was going and he wasn't. Tula kissed her goodbye and went into the room to cry. Charlie told her to get in the car before she changed her mind. She got in, and they left.

When they got to Georgia, she called to let us know they made it. It only took four hours. All the kids wanted to speak to her, and so did everybody else. Mama told her to call at least once a week. They didn't have their own phone. They used their neighbor's.

It was a month before they got a chance to come home. Charlie had to catch up on bills. Whenever Gent called, she'd tell Mama about how bad she wanted to come home.

Mama told her not to be worrying Charlie about coming home because he had other bills and that some of us would go see her when we could. She was just like a spoiled child.

She would just say, "I wanna see y'all now. I don't wanna wait till some other time. I wanna come home now."

When they did come home, Gent had gained a lot of weight. It looked like somebody had taken an air pump and blown her up. None of us complained because we felt lucky to have her around.

Mama said, "Lord, you fat. And thank the Lord for that. How ya feelin'?"

"I feel fine. Better than I have in a long time."

"I gotta tell Hannah to come and take a look atcha. I know she ain't gon' believe it when she see ya."

Aunt Kitty came over when she saw them getting out of the car. "Hey, sweetheart." She hugged Gent and kissed her on the cheek. "Ya sho lookin' good."

"No, I ain't either. I look like a pig."

"Well, be thankful. Ya could've not been here at all."

"Oh, I am. You can believe that."

They came in the house out of the cold, and the kids were all over her. Aunt Kitty was bringing Ricky in, and she kissed him.

THE FIRST CASE OF LUPUS

When Gent got by the heater, she said, "I thought Ricky would worry me to death."

Mama said, "About what?"

"Wantin' to come home. Every five minutes, he was sayin' that he wanted to go home. Now that he here, he can stay."

Mama laughed and hugged Ricky.

Aunt Kitty said, "I'm glad he ain't goin' back maself."

Then Tula and Von started yelling and jumping up and down, saying, "I wanna go! I wanna go!"

Mama told both of them to hush 'cause neither one of them was going back.

They went to see all of our aunts while they were home.

When they first saw Gent, they all said the same thing, "Lord, you fat. Ya look good though."

Aunt Kitty went with them. She'd ride whenever she got a chance. Aunt Hannah told her that she had said a prayer for her every night since she left and that she knew they were answered because the Lord had brought her back from the grave. Essie told her that she had been knocking on death's door, but he just wouldn't open it.

When they got back to the house, Gent decided to take Von with her. Tula got mad. Mama told her that she couldn't go because of school. She didn't care. She wanted to go anyway.

That Sunday evening, they left. We waited long enough for them to get there before we expected a call. Six hours after they left, we still hadn't heard anything. At twelve o'clock that night, the phone rang. It was Gent.

The first thing Mama asked her was "What took ya so long to call?"

"We just gettin' here. We had a little bit of car trouble."

"How did ya get it fixed?"

"A highway patrolman stopped to see what the problem was, and he went and got a tow truck to pull us to a service station, and they fixed it there."

"Oh, what was wrong wit it?"

"Somethin' had to do wit the radiator."

"Well, I can go to sleep now. I was waitin' for ya to call and let me know y'all made it."

"Yeah, we made it. I ain't gonna call back till the end of the week. I go for ma checkup tomorrow."

"All right, I'll talk to ya then."

"Okay, see ya later."

"All right," Mama said. Then she went to sleep.

Gent waited till I got home from school before she called.

When the phone rang, Mama hollered from the kitchen, "That's probably Gent. I was waitin' for her to call."

Sterling and I ran to the phone. I beat him to it, and he got mad and started calling me names. I laughed at him and answered the phone.

"Hey, where Mama?"

"In the kitchen. You comin' home this week?"

"I doubt if we'll make it this weekend. Since Christmas is the week after, we might wait till then. How you and Rabbit doin'?"

"Fine, child. Is Von ready to come home yet?"

"Yeah, but he'll sho have to wait. Put Mama on the phone."

I called her to come and get it.

"Hey, what did the doctor say?"

"I'm doin' fine. I don't have to take as much medicine now. He cut me back some. I only take two prednisones. I'm glad too. He said that that's what got me swole up like this."

"That's good. Ya gotta be doin' all right for him to do that."

"He said that I was. Now I'ma put maself on a diet."

"A diet! Ain't cha been po' long enough?"

"I said I'ma go on a diet, not starvation."

Mama laughed. "Sarah said that, if she knew you was home, she woulda came by here to see ya and said for you to come and see her the next time ya come home."

"Tell her that I sho will. Let me speak to the kids and JD before I hang up. I don't wanna run ya bill up too high."

Mama called them to the phone. She said hi to all of them and told Sterling to put me back on the phone for a minute.

THE FIRST CASE OF LUPUS

He handed me the phone and said, "Here, buzzard," then dropped it on the chair.

She said, "Charlie got a friend that sell reefer, and, girl, the stuff is good."

I said, "Whatcha tellin' me for? I can't get none of it."

"That's what I wanted to speak to ya again for. I'ma send ya a couple of joints in ma next letter."

"Okay. I'll be lookin' for it. You can bring some home witcha when ya come the next time."

"Don't worry. I am."

Mama hollered and told me to hang up 'cause we had already ran the phone bill up enough for one day. I told Gent bye and hung up.

When they came home for Christmas, Gent had lost a lot of weight. When we were alone, I asked her how she lost weight so fast.

"Takin' speckled birds."

"You ain't scared to take 'em bein' as sick as you was?"

"Nope. But I got to ease up on 'em 'cause they startin' to make me feel nervous in the stomach. Don't tell Mama or Aunt Kitty that I'm takin' 'em. They'll have a fit."

"I won't. How do they make ya feel?"

"Ya feel high a little bit. But ya don't have no kinda appetite."

"The doctor told you that you could take 'em?"

"No. I'ma quit 'cause I'm back down to the size I wanted to be."

Randy came out of the house asking Charlie to take him for a ride in his mean Chevy.

Charlie said, "I'm just about ready to trade that shit."

"Ain't nobody gon' give you no car for that piece of shit. You might as well take it up there to Grim's and sell it for junk."

They started laughing.

"No, I'll try to trade it first. I might trade it while I'm home."

"Ya might as well 'cause it look like it can't stand another trip back to Georgia."

"If I don't trade it, I'ma leave it here with Gent for her to get around."

Randy looked over at Gent. "Bummer ain't goin' back?"

"Not right now. Them damn people we rentin' from wanna shoot the rent up to two hundred a month. We ain't payin' but one twenty-five now."

"Them mothers tryin' to get greedy."

"Damn right. So I told Gent to stay until I find us another place, then I'll come back and get her."

"I know she was glad to hear that."

"Shine yeah. You shoulda seen her clappin' her hands. It didn't matter to her that they took the rent up. She said they shoulda did it sooner. That girl know she don't like it down there. She said that's redneck country."

"I bet them some damn fools down there too."

"They try to be."

"Let's ride over to Deb's. I would drive my car, but I ain't got no gas."

"All right," said Charlie, and they left.

Charlie had to be back the day after Christmas. Gent and I took him to the bus station.

He told Gent, "I'll let ya know when I find us a place."

She said, "Don't be in no hurry."

He laughed and said, "Yo' ole ass think you funny."

He kissed her goodbye.

Three weeks later, he called and said that he had found another trailer and that he'd be home the weekend to get her. She said okay, and after she got off the phone, she started getting their stuff together. He called back on Friday and said that he had to pull guard duty all weekend and told her to ask Randy if he would bring her down there.

She said, "I'll ask him. What we gonna do about the gas and stuff?"

"Tell him to put it in, and I'll give him the money back. Ya turn off on Exit 7. When ya turn off, they'll be a Holiday Inn on ya left. That's where I'll be waitin' for y'all at. I'll give y'all five hours."

"That's if that ole car don't give us any trouble. Let me ask him before ya hang up." She went into his room and asked him. "Randy, Charlie told me to ask you if you would take me to Georgia. He woulda came home, but he got guard duty this weekend."

THE FIRST CASE OF LUPUS

"Yeah. We can leave in the mornin' after I get off work. What about the gas and oil? That car usin' oil bad as hell."

"He said that, if you put it in, he'll pay you back as soon as we get there."

"All right."

She went back to the phone and told him what Randy said.

He said, "Wait till about eleven or twelve before y'all leave so I'll be off and can meetcha."

"Okay. I'll see ya tomorrow. Bye."

Mama asked her, "Who ya gonna take to stay witcha this time?"

"I don't really need nobody now. I can stay by maself."

"All right. If ya get lonely or start feelin' bad, call me, and somebody'll go stay witcha."

"Don't worry. I will."

The next day at eleven thirty, they left. Randy got Lester to ride with them. He filled up with gas and got a half a case of oil. They didn't get there until nine that night because they had car trouble, but Charlie was still there waiting for them. Randy and Lester didn't get back until the next day at six. They had to go to work that night. When he told Charlie about the car and how bad it was running, he said that the next time he hit Dillon, he was going straight to the car dealer and get him another one.

A week passed without us hearing anything from Gent. That made Mama worry. The next day, she called.

Mama said, "Why you ain't call me before now?"

"I was doin' all right, so I just didn't call. I didn't wanna run up ya phone bill for nothin'."

"Didn't I tell ya to call me once a week?"

"That's true. But I know you hate to have a lotta bills too."

"Don't worry about that. You just call me once a week like I told ya."

"All right."

"How Charlie doin'?"

"Fine. How is everybody there?"

"Just fine. When you'll be home?"

"I don't know yet. Charlie been workin' every weekend since I been here."

"Well, long as ya doin' good, don't worry him about comin'."

"I ain't. Well, I'ma go get back to this house so I can cook. Lord, the girl that live next door to me will talk ya to death."

"At least she'll keep ya company. Is she Black or White?"

"Black and big and fat."

Mama laughed and said, "I'ma go 'cause I already got pots on."

"Okay, I'll call ya back this weekend if nothin' don't happen."

"All right, bye."

The next morning, when Gent woke up, something didn't seem right. She knew she had both of her eyes open, but she could only see out of one.

"Charlie. Charlie, wake up."

He woke up and turned to her.

"Is this eye open?" she said.

He said, "Yeah. Why?"

"I can't see out of it."

He sat up in the bed and said, "Whatcha mean ya can't see out of it?"

"Just like I said! I can't see out of it!"

Charlie jumped up and grabbed his pants. "Try not to get upset. Put on ya clothes, and let's go see a doctor. I'll call in and tell 'em that I need the day off."

Gent started crying and saying, "Lord, please don't let me go blind. Let anything else happen, but don't let me go blind, please."

Charlie went to her and hugged her. "Don't think like that. It might just be somethin' that'll clear up. We have to hope so anyway."

"But what if it don't?" She sat down on the bed and put her face in her hands and cried. "Lord, what did I do wrong to deserve this?"

"Wait and see what the doctor say before ya run ya blood back up again, okay? He should be able to tell us somethin'. Go on and finish puttin' on ya clothes."

She couldn't help but cry. Slowly she managed to put on her clothes. Charlie asked her if she wanted him to help her, but she said no and that she could do it. He took her to the doctor, and they had

THE FIRST CASE OF LUPUS

to wait about thirty minutes before he saw her. He checked both eyes with a small light. He told her that she was completely blind in her right eye and there was nothing to be done to help it. He told her the left eye was fine, but she'd have to get treatment for her eyes.

She asked him, "Where is the closest eye clinic at?"

He said, "There's one in Charleston, South Carolina, and there's also one in California. The one in Charleston would be a lot closer."

"Is there any way you could set up me an appointment?"

"Yes, ma'am. Can you make it this coming Monday? You should start the treatment as soon as possible."

"Yeah, I believe I can make it."

"All right, Mrs. Taylor. I'll have my nurse to make it. I'll be seeing you."

"All right, thank you."

As soon as they left, Gent had Charlie find a pay phone. She wanted to tell Mama what had happened.

Mama said, "Do ya want me to come down there and stay witcha for a while? I can get Kitty to stay here if ya do."

"I wouldn't mind it. Me and Charlie was talkin', and he said that Yolanda, the girl that stay next to me, could take me in our car."

"When ya gotta be there?"

"Monday mornin'. Can ya be here by then?"

"Yeah. Meet me at the bus station Sunday evenin'."

"Okay."

"All right then. Talk to ya later." Mama hung up and told us about what had happened to Gent.

Mama arrived in Georgia around ten that night. Charlie was waiting for her, but Gent stayed at home.

She said, "Gent didn't feel like comin'?"

"She home cookin'."

"Cookin'! This time a' night? Her eye must not be botherin' her?"

"It don't hurt her or nothin'. She just can't see out of it."

"Oh. Well, that's good. Which one is it she can't see out of?"

"I believe it's the right one."

"What they say caused it?"

"That sickness she got."

"I thought she was over that?"

"They said she'll never get over it. It's gon' be there for life. It's one of the effects of it."

Gent had to go to Charleston every day for a week to get laser beams shot in her eye. It wasn't painful, but she still didn't like having that done to her. The only reason she was doing it was that she didn't want to go blind. She always complained about having to take that ride every day.

Mama said, "Child, you ought to sit down somewhere and hush. You should thank the Lord for not takin' both of 'em."

"I do, but I still hate goin' over there every day."

"Well, maybe after this week ya won't have to go every day."

"I sho hope not. Then maybe I can go home for a while. If ya ready to go back after this week, I might go too."

"Charlie ain't gon' letcha go nowhere."

"Yes, he will. If you leave, he ain't gonna have no other way to take me to Charleston. He ain't gonna let big Yodi take me 'cause she drive like a race-car driver." She laughed as she said it.

When they got home that night, they talked to Charlie about it. He decided to let Gent come back home with Mama. She finished her treatment for the week and asked them if she had to come every day like always. They told her no, and they would set her an appointment for once a week. She had to go back the following Wednesday.

She called home and said that they'd be leaving Saturday morning and should be home by five thirty that evening. Charlie told her, if she needed anything, to let him know. She told him that he didn't have to worry about that because he'd be the first to know.

The next day, Cookie and I went to the bus station to get them. We met them as they got off the bus. We had to wait about ten minutes to get her bags and boxes. After we got them and put them in the car, the first thing Gent said was that she wanted to go to Deb's house and get her a bag.

Mama said, "Lord have mercy."

We didn't stay long when we got there. Mama didn't get out of the car, so we knew that she was ready to get home. Deb wanted to

THE FIRST CASE OF LUPUS

ask Gent about what had happened, but she said that she'd come over to the house and talk.

When we got home Aunt Kitty and Randy had all kinds of questions for her. She said that Aunt Essie called and wanted her to call her back as soon as she got there. She was ready to come home again if anybody needed her. Mama told her that it was all right.

Cookie, Gent, and I went on the patio and talked while we waited for Deb to come. Cookie told us that she didn't think she was going to graduate. She asked Gent if she could go stay with her when she went back to Georgia. She said that she didn't care. Gent asked her if Mama knew that she wasn't going to graduate. She said no. Gent asked her why, and she said that she was scared.

Gent asked her, "Scared of what?"

"They lookin' for me to finish. I hate to tell them that I ain't, especially after what all they did for me."

"The only thing she'll probably say is that school won't be meant for everybody."

"Well, you talk to her then. If I go back wit you, I might get ma a job."

"Yeah, you might. And she don't want me to be by maself anyway."

"That's right. So she might not mind it too much. I hope not anyway."

"Don't worry about it. I'll talk to her."

I was sitting there getting a little jealous. I wanted to go and stay with her myself, but I knew that I couldn't because I was still in school.

Mama tried to get her to stay, but Gent knew that Charlie wouldn't go for that. So Mama asked her if she was going to take one of the kids back with her.

She said, "I know for sho that Ricky ain't goin' back. Cookie said that she would go because she don't think that she gonna graduate."

"She don't? She didn't tell me that, and Kitty ain't say nothin' about it."

"She scared to tell y'all. I told her that she could if it was okay wit y'all."

"Well, if she ain't gonna graduate, she might as well go on and give up. That way, you'll have somebody there witcha."

"She wanna find her a job down there. That way, she'll have her own money."

Then Mama asked her if she was going to let her mom know about it.

Gent said, "I reckon she will, but we gonna see how things turn out first."

Wednesday came, and Randy and Deb took her for her treatment. They drove Mama's Plymouth. It took them three hours to get there. All of them were getting high and enjoying the ride.

Randy asked Gent, "Do you know how to get to the place?"

"After I get in Charleston, I can almost take ya right to the place. I can't tell ya where to go until we get off the main road. The way we goin' in now is from a different way we came from Georgia."

"Don't worry about it. We'll get there."

Deb said, "Yeah, all of us together should be able to find it, right?"

Randy and Gent agreed with her.

When they got there, they walked in with her, went to check and see if her name was on the list, and waited with her until they called her; and then they got up and left. They went walking to find a store and get a few beers. Deb said that they had to get some more weed because they smoked all she had on the way there.

They were in luck.

Some guy walked up to them with a funny accent and said, "Me got some good green."

Randy asked, "How ya sellin' it?"

"Whatever you want, me got it."

"Give me a nickel."

Deb said, "Get a dime. I got the other half on it."

Randy gave the guy $10 for the weed, and they left. They went to the car and smoked a couple of joints.

"Damn if this ain't a good dime. And it's good too. It got me fucked up," said Deb.

"You ain't by yo'self."

THE FIRST CASE OF LUPUS

"We shoulda got two of them. I bet we couldn't find him now for hell."

"Hell no. That ugly mug look like he was on the move," Deb said, and they started laughing. "Ya reckon they called Gent yet?"

"I don't know. Ya wanna go see?"

"Yeah, let's walk some. If I sit here much longer, I'll go to sleep."

They got out and went into the clinic where Gent was. They grinned and talked about people all the way in. Deb went up to the desk and asked the nurse if they had called Gent yet. She told her that they had.

When Deb got back to her seat, Randy said, "Whatcha go ask that woman that for? You didn't see her out here, so you know they had to call her back there."

Both of them started laughing again. Both of them had deep voices, and you could hear them over the whole waiting room.

Then Randy said, "Let's go find somethin' to drink."

They left.

The doctor started the treatment. They took her to a small room and turned off the lights. They had these little, tiny flashlights looking in her eyes. They shot the laser beams in her eyes and some drops. She had to sit there for a minute until some of her vision returned. The nurse led her back out to the lobby. Randy got up and met her and took her by the arm.

He said, "Can ya see?"

"Yeah, a little bit. Don't turn me loose."

"I ain't."

"Do it hurt?" asked Deb.

"No. Everything's just blurry."

They got in the car and left.

Deb asked her, "Do ya feel too bad to smoke a joint?"

"No, not if ya got one."

Randy laughed and said, "Ya know that eye won't botherin' her bad enough to turn down a joint."

Gent said, "You ain't lyin'."

"What did they do to it?" asked Deb.

"Shot some mo' laser beams in it. I'll be glad when I get through wit that mess too."

"So you gonna have to come back again for mo'?"

"When?" asked Randy.

"Next week at the same time."

"So you ain't goin' back to Georgia?"

"No, not right now anyway."

"Well, you don't mind it too much, do ya?" asked Deb.

"Girl, you know I don't. You'll bring me back, Randy?"

"Yeah. Who else gon' bring ya?"

Deb said, "If I don't have anything else to do, I'ma come back too."

When they got back home, Gent called Charlie and told him that she wasn't going to go back right then.

He said, "Why? They got to keep givin' ya that stuff?"

"Yeah, once a week. My next appointment is next week at the same time like today. I figured that it would be too much ridin' for me to go all the way back down there and have to come back here. It would save some money too. Don't cha think?"

"Yep. You can come for a weekend, can't cha? Or either I come home, one."

"Either way. Whichever way ya wanna do it, let me know."

"Okay. I got to go now, but I'ma call ya maybe Friday."

"Okay. Love ya. Bye."

The days seemed to go by quickly. When Joe found out Gent was home, he came by every day and night trying to get her to go off with him, but she wouldn't. He would ask me to help him get her. I'd pretend to go along with him and tell her what he'd say. We'd laugh, and she wouldn't pay either of us any attention.

We sat up late the night before she had to go back to Charleston. She was telling us about what the doctor had said about trying a new way of treating her eye.

"He said that it won't gonna hurt, but I betcha it will," said Gent.

Cookie said, "Ya scared, ain't cha?"

THE FIRST CASE OF LUPUS

"I believe I'm makin' ma ownself scared just wonderin' what he gonna do to me."

"Yep," said Cookie. "And ya don't even know what he gonna do yet."

"I don't know, but if it hurt too bad, I won't be goin' back for no mo'."

I said, "Don't say that now. You'll go back if ya don't wanna go blind."

Gent decided to call Deb to see if she was still going to go. The phone rang a few times before she answered. She told Gent that she wouldn't be able to make it and for her to catch her the next time.

Gent said, "I sho wish you could go wit me tomorrow, Head."

I said, "I'll go."

"Mama ain't gonna say nothin', ya reckon?"

"No. I ain't got no tests or nothin', and I ain't missed but 'bout three or four days out of school."

"Well, gawn and ask her now then and see what she say."

I went in the room and asked her. It was just like I thought it would be. She said that she didn't care and that it was up to me. Then I went to bed so that I could be ready the next morning when Randy got home from work.

We left as soon as he got home. We stopped at a gas station and gassed up and had the oil checked. We talked all the way there. Randy was trying to listen to what we were talking about and missed his turn. Before he realized it, we were almost in Conway.

We were still talking when Randy said, "I'll be damn. I missed ma turn. That's what I get for tryin' to listen to everything y'all talkin' asses sayin'."

Gent said, "Well, hell. We didn't tell ya to listen. That was you bein' nosy, not wantin' to miss nothin'."

I said, "That's right. You didn't have to listen."

Randy, always being a nasty mouth, said, "Shut the fuck up, both of ya."

We laughed.

Then he said, "Y'all worry the hell out of me. From here on out till we get there, just shutcha damn mouths, all right?"

Both of us said, "It ain't our fault. You the one drivin'."

"I swear. Sixty miles off track. If this ain't a damn shame."

I said, "Well, don't blame me. I didn't come witcha the first time, so I don't know where you supposed to turn at."

When we got back on the right road, he said, "Y'all can start talkin' again now. I know where I'm at."

We had not stopped.

We waited fifteen minutes before they called her. When they did, I went with her to get her treatment.

On the way back there, she said, "I didn't think thatcha was gonna come wit me. I'm glad ya did 'cause I ain't never had this done that they gon' do today."

"I wanna see how they gon' do it."

"Last week, I asked Debra Jean if she was gonna come back here wit me, and she said no."

"I didn't wanna sit out there in that waitin' room all that time."

"Randy still out there?"

"No. As I was leavin' to catch up wit you, he got up and said that he was goin' to the car and go to sleep."

A nurse came by in the hallway where we were standing and told Gent to go in the room right in front of us. I went in with her. It must have been all right because she didn't tell me to leave or anything.

A few minutes later, the doctor came in. "Hi, Jeanette. How are you doing today?"

"Fine, and you?"

"Okay. You remember last week I told you that we were going to try freezing your eye to see how that would work?"

"Yes, I remember."

"It's going to hurt just a little bit. It'll feel about like a mosquito bite. What I'm going to do is give you a shot on each side of your eyeball. Then I'm going to take this little instrument and freeze the whole eyeball."

Gent put her face in her hands and started shaking her head.

"It's not as bad as it sounds. You'll only feel a little sting, okay?"

"All right, whatever you say."

THE FIRST CASE OF LUPUS

"Are you ready? And do you have any questions?"

"Yes. My sister can stay in here with me, can't she?"

"Yes, she sure can."

Gent got into the chair that looked like a barber's chair. He told her to relax, and he reclined the chair back. He turned out all the lights and had one small one that looked like a little spotlight. It shined only on her face. He picked up a needle and told Gent to look over to her left. When she did, he took the needle and stuck it in the right side next to the eyeball. Gent was lifting her body up off the chair like somebody had their arms under her and was picking her up. He kept telling her to be as still as possible. Then he told her to look to her right. He gave her another shot in the eye.

He told her that it wouldn't hurt, but from the way she was coming up out of that chair, she had to be feeling something. It wasn't until he started freezing it that she hollered out.

She kept saying, "Oh, it's hurtin'."

The doctor would just say, "I'm just about finished, Jeanette."

He did it a little while longer, then he told her to lie back for a little while and then she could go.

After he left out, Gent said, "Lord have mercy. I don't think I can go through that again. That man told me that it won't gon' hurt. That's the biggest lie he ever told."

"I don't think I coulda stood it with him stickin' me in the eye like that."

"This whole side of ma face feel numb."

The doctor came back in and told her that she could go. He told her, if she happened to start aching, to take a Tylenol or aspirin and lie down. I had to practically lead her to the car. On our way out, they called me back to get her slip for her next appointment.

She grunted all the way to the car and kept complaining about her face feeling numb.

When we got to the car, she told me to get in the front. She wanted to get in the back so she could lie down.

The first few miles out of Charleston, she kept moaning.

Randy asked her, "Ya want me to stop and getcha somethin' to take?"

"Yeah. Get me a Goody's Powder. Get me a ginger ale to take it with too."

He went into the store. He brought back what I wanted so I could stay in the car with Gent.

She took the Goody's Powder, but it didn't do her any good. She only got worse. Before we got halfway home, she was crying and holding her head.

She was saying, "Lord, I can't stand this pain. I can't stand it."

I'd look back at her. I knew there was nothing I could do but feel sorry for her. I would look at Randy.

Then he'd ask her if she wanted him to stop and get her something else for her head.

She said, "Yeah. Get me two more packs of Goody's Powder."

I said, "Ya gonna take both of 'em?"

"Yep."

When Randy got back with them, she said, "If these don't stop it, ya won't have to stop no mo'."

"Don't worry 'bout that. If ya need 'em, I don't mind stoppin'."

After taking all four of those, the pain still got worse. They got so bad that the only thing she could do was lie there and moan.

Once in a while, we could hear her say, "Oh, Lord, have mercy. Oh, I'm hurtin'."

She moaned and groaned all the way home. We felt so sorry for her that, for a long time, we rode without saying a word.

All of a sudden, she got quiet. All we could hear was the motor of the car. I looked back at Gent and asked her if she might feel a little better sittin' up. She didn't say anything right then, so I asked her again.

She waited a few seconds and said, "No. I'll try it later."

"It musta eased off some?"

"A little bit."

Randy said, "Don't make her talk. That might start it to hurtin' bad again."

So I stopped talking to her and started talking to him.

Thirty-three miles before we got home, Gent started having sharp pains in her head again. She told Randy that she had to have

THE FIRST CASE OF LUPUS

something. He stopped at the next store and got her a bottle of extra-strength Tylenol. They cost him $7.95. He complained about the price, but he got them anyway. She told me to open them for her and to hand her two of them.

"You don't think all that medicine you took gon' make you sick on the stomach?" I asked.

"If it stop this pain, I don't care about it makin' me sick."

"Well, between them six Goody's Powders and those two Tylenols, it should stop somethin' from hurtin'."

Randy said, "You ain't lyin'."

It didn't help any though. When we got home, it was almost dark. Bobby came up at the same time we did. We were out of the car, and I was helping Gent out. By the time I got her out, Randy and Bobby each grabbed one of her arms and helped her into the house. Mama held the door open for them. She told them to take her to her room. Mama helped her take off her clothes and put her to bed. She cried half of the night, but when she went to sleep, she slept till the middle of the next day.

Mama went into her room at eleven thirty to check on her. "How ya head doin' this mornin'? It ain't hurtin', is it?"

"I can feel a little pain in it, but it ain't as bad as it was yesterday."

"I put ya Tylenols right there by ya bed. I'll send for some Goody's Powders if ya want some."

"I'll try these for a while and see how they do me."

"What did they do this time to make ya hurt so bad? You ain't been hurtin' like that."

"They froze this eye. They had to give me two shots in my eyeball."

"Oh, Jesus! If I'da seen that, I woulda passed out."

"I thought I was gonna mess all over myself. I started comin' out that chair they had me sittin' in. Ole Head stayed in there wit me the whole time."

"That was good. You couldn't see when ya first came out, could ya?"

"No. Nothin'. Head had to lead me to the car."

"When ya next appointment?"

"He want me to go back next month, but if it's gon' make me hurt like it did this time, I'd rather not go back."

"Well, ya better go. Ya know that's for ya own good. When ya gon' call Charlie?"

"He gonna call me. I know he gonna want me to come home."

"Well, you won't be there by yaself. You still takin' Cookie witcha, ain't cha?"

"Yeah, if she still wanna go."

"She said she was."

"Well, when Cookie go back with me, then who gonna stay with Aunt Kitty?"

"Na said that he was gonna stay with her."

"Oh."

Charlie called, and he decided to come and get Gent that coming weekend. She didn't want to go, but she went because Charlie wanted her to. Cookie was all excited about going. She hardly ever went anywhere, and this was one trip that she was looking forward to. We hated to see her go again. Mama told her the same thing each time she left, and that was to call her once a week.

It was a month before they came home again, but we heard from them every week. Cookie found a job at a sewing plant, and Gent told me that she thought she might be pregnant. I told her that I thought that I was too.

We didn't say anything about it to Mama or Aunt Kitty.

We wanted to be sure before we told them. Gent said they were going to be home the last weekend of this month, which was May, and we could to the clinic together for the tests. I told her okay, and she hung up.

I had two weeks to wait for Gent. When they did finally get home, I thought they were only going to stay a weekend, but they came for a week. I should have known that because they gave pregnancy test only on Wednesdays. Wednesday, we went to take them, and they cost $6 each. Both of our tests came back positive.

When Gent came out of the office, she came to me and said, "They told me it was positive. What do that mean?"

THE FIRST CASE OF LUPUS

I said, "That mean thatcha pregnant, fool. You should know that. You got three kids already."

"But, girl, it's been six years since I had to do anything like this."

"That don't make no difference. I wonder what Bobby Gene gonna say?"

"I don't know about him, but Charlie gon' be happy. I told him that I thought I was. That's why he was so willin' for me to come home and see."

When we left the clinic, we went to Deb's. When she heard the news about us, she started joking and saying there were going to be two big mamas in the family.

When Gent and Cookie went back to Georgia, it was a while before they came home again. With Gent's pregnancy, she didn't want to do too much traveling.

After we got into some months of pregnancy, the doctor told Gent that she wasn't supposed to be able to conceive any more kids because of her sickness. That proved to be wrong. He kept a close eye on her because of all the medication she was taking for her condition. They warned her that it could be harmful to the baby.

I worked in tobacco that summer, and the last week of finishing for the year, I saved my money and told Bobby that I wanted to go see Gent. He said okay. After he got off of work, he got him a couple of hours of sleep, picked up his cousin Chester, and came and got me and Sterling. We had a good time on the ride there. We got there around seven that evening. They were glad to see us. Gent asked us if we wanted anything to eat. We said no because we had stopped on the way and got something. We sat around and played cards.

She looked at me and said, "Hey, Head, you sure you ain't gotcha time mixed up? You look like ya 'bout ready to have li'l Rabbit."

That's what they called Bobby, Rabbit.

Chester laughed. "She sho do, don't she? When you suppose to have yours?"

"Me and her supposed to be together."

Charlie said, "Y'all sho don't look like it. Head ain't gon' make it till December."

Bobby said, "You ain't lyin'. Look like she ready now."

Everybody laughed.

"I know when I'ma have my baby. I ain't thinkin' 'bout none of ya," I said.

Cookie came and rubbed my stomach. "Come on and go to the store with me. We can walk if you want to," she said.

Charlie said, "Ya see the name of the store, don't cha? Get and Go. That's just what they wantcha to do, get and go."

Bobby said, "Shit?"

"I ain't lyin', man. Look out the window. You can see it from here. No car stay too long."

He got up and looked out the window. "I swear it is, ain't it?"

"Yeah. They don't wantcha to hang around none. When ya go to use the phone, they be lookin' atcha like they readin' ya lips."

"Well, I ain't gonna be in there long enough for 'em to know that I was there," I said.

"Hurry back so we can play some Spades."

"Y'all got enough to get started. You ain't got to wait on us."

"Just do what I said and hurry back. I ain't played witcha in a good while, and I wanna see if ya still know how."

"I can play better than you."

"You wish," said Charlie.

Cookie and I left and went to the store. They didn't miss us.

We played Spades for hours. The guys went to the store and got some beer. Yoddi had come over, and we were still playing while they were gone. It was then that I found out just how much Yoddi could talk. She went on and on the whole time we played.

The night went by quickly. The next day, we got up and ate breakfast. Bobby said that we would leave at ten so that he would have time to get him some sleep for work that night. We sat around and talked, and before we left, she was asking us when we would be back again. Bobby said that he didn't know. I told her that I would be back as soon as I could. I was gonna catch the next ride coming her way.

At ten, we left. The ride didn't seem as long as it had on the way there. When I got home, everybody was asking how Gent was doing. Mama told Randy that she wanted to go the week after next. He said okay.

Then Mama looked at me and said, "Do you know the way back to her house?"

"Yeah. Ya don't have to make but 'bout two turns, and ya there."

"I don't want her to know that we comin'. But we gon' have to go before school start back."

"Yep. I'll take ya right to the front door."

Randy said, "We'll sho go. I gotta get ma car checked out."

"I'll get Kitty to stay here wit the children when we go."

"Oh yeah. Wit Silver Jean goin', I won't have to do all the drivin'."

"How ya figure?" I asked.

"Girl, you know damn well you can help me drive. Bobby Gene didn't do all the drivin' by hisself, did he?"

"What that got to do with it?"

"Nothin', but you gon' help me drive."

"Yeah, she gonna help ya," Mama said.

The case was closed because what Mama says goes.

Those two weeks went by like the wind. Deb had told us that she wanted to go with us. On our way out, we went by and picked her up. Randy's little Camaro could only hold four people. The kids wanted to go, but there wasn't enough room.

When we got to Gent's house, they weren't there. Randy and Deb went around back to see if they could find a way in.

Mama said, "Y'all know that y'all ain't gonna be able to get in. I bet she got everything locked up."

A few minutes later, Mama and I heard them walking through the house.

When they opened the door, Randy said, "Tell me I can't find a way in here. We got in, didn't we?"

"Y'all could go to jail for breakin' and enterin'," Mama said and started laughing.

"It won't that hard to get in. All we did was fumble with the doorknob, and it popped open."

"I got to tell 'em about that. They need to get it fixed if it's that easy to open," said Mama.

Deb said, "I wish that we could hide the car. That way, she won't know we here."

Mama said, "No, don't hide the car. The po' child might come home and be scared to come into her own house. She'll think somebody broke in and waitin' for 'em to come back."

"Her and Charlie must be gone grocery shoppin' 'cause there sho ain't nothin' in here," I said, looking in the refrigerator.

"They'll probably be back after a while."

Deb said, "Let's walk out here to the store and call to the house to see if she called."

Randy and I said all right, and we left.

On the way, I said, "Check out the name of this store."

"Get and Go. Damn, they don't mean for nobody to hang around, do they?" asked Randy while Deb was on the phone calling home.

Randy and I went in and got something with which to make some sandwiches. When we came out, she was talking to Na. She started laughing.

Randy said, "What he talkin' 'bout?"

"He said that we was gonna go to jail down here breakin' in somebody house around all these rednecks."

Randy said, "Gent and Charlie ain't gonna let 'em take us to jail. Did she call them?"

"No." Then she told Na, "Well, let us get back to the house. I wanna be there when she come."

Na said, "Tell Randy that I didn't think that his little Camaro was gonna make it one time."

Deb laughed and told him what Na said.

He said, "Tell Na to go to hell."

Na laughed and said, "I heard that, fool. I'll see ya later."

While we were at her house, she was at a phone booth calling home.

Na answered the phone. "Hello."

THE FIRST CASE OF LUPUS

"Collect call from Jeanette Taylor. Will you accept the call?" the operator said.

"Yeah."

"Hey, where Mama?"

"At yo' house."

"No, they ain't. I just left home."

"Well, they in the wrong damn house then. They just called and said that they got in the house some kinda way."

"Who came with her besides Randy?"

"Silver Jean and Debra Jean."

"Who there with you?"

"Aunt Kitty and the children."

"Let me speak to her before I go."

He gave Aunt Kitty the phone.

"Hi, baby, how ya doin'?"

"Just fine. I wanted to speak to ya before I go back home."

"Ya won't lookin' for ya mama to come this week, was ya?"

"No, I sho won't. Why she didn't call and let me know that she was comin'?"

"She asked Silver Jean did she know the way back to ya house, and she said yeah. So Nank wanted to surprise ya by comin' and not lettin' ya know. They just called a few minutes ago. Randy said him and Deb found a way in by the back door."

Both of them started laughing.

"Well, let me go. I'll talk to ya later."

"Okay. Take care of yaself. Bye."

When they got back home, we were listening to music and eating sandwiches.

Gent said, "I'll be dog if this don't beat it all."

Mama said, "I was hopin' that y'all would be here when we got here. I said, 'Lord, we gon' have to sit in the car and wait for 'em.' Randy and Debra Jean got out and went 'round the house, and when I looked again, they was comin' out the front door."

Gent looked at me and said, "Ole Head brought y'all right to the front door."

"Right to it."

"I didn't think ya could find ya way back after just one time comin'."

I said, "It won't that hard. When we was leavin', I told Bobby Gene that I believed I could come back without anybody showin' me."

Randy said, "I can too. Ya don't have to make but two turns."

"I'm sho glad to see y'all. How'd y'all get that there to come?" asked Gent, looking at Deb.

Deb said, "Whatcha mean? I ain't gotta stay home all the time."

Mama said, "Where Trica?"

"She got her ole dumbass over there at Yodi house. She been over there for the last two days. She mad with me and Charlie. She told Yodi that we was tryin' to use her just because we asked her to help out with the bills and stuff."

"What she think? That she gonna stay here for nothin'? If she can't stay here witcha like she supposed to, then she might as well come on back home. She don't know enough about that girl to be stayin' wit her. Is she over there now?"

"No. I think they gone uptown."

"Well, when she get back, I'ma have a talk with that sister."

"We'll know when they get back 'cause nosy Yodi gonna have to come and see who drivin' that car out there."

"Who car? Randy's?"

"Yeah."

"Is she that nosy, girl?" asked Deb.

"Girl, yeah."

Randy said, "Is she got any money?"

"Shit no," Charlie said. "She don't do nothin' but sit over there in that house and mind other peoples' business."

"Wait till ya see her. You wouldn't want her even if she had any. Her husband tickle me. He said that, when he first saw Yodi, she was at a club with a big fur jacket on, diamond rings on her fingers, and spendin' big money. He married her and found out that she didn't have shit."

"And Trica believe everything she say," Charlie said.

"Lord, I can't wait to meet her," Deb said.

THE FIRST CASE OF LUPUS

We saw a car pull up in the yard next door, and it was them. She didn't even take time to go in the house when she got out of the car. She came right over to Gent's. She gave Trica the keys so that she could get in.

I opened the door before she got to it and told Trica that Mama wanted to see her. She said okay and she would be there in a minute. Yodi came on in and started talking as soon as she hit the door. She looked like she weighed a good 350 pounds.

She walked in and said, "Hi, Ms. Casey, it's good to see ya again. I know Gent's glad to see ya. All of y'all that don't know me, I'm Yolanda, but everybody call me Yodi. And, oh, you must be Randy! I feel like I already know you from listenin' to Trica and Gent talkin' about cha. And yo' name is?"

"Debra."

"Yep, Debra Jean. I feel like I know all of y'all. I thought y'all mighta been playin' Spades."

"We can play a hand if ya wanna," said Gent.

"Yeah, child. I'ma have to go cook Billy somethin' to eat though later on. He'll be home by six thirty."

Then Trica walked in.

She said, "Be my partner, Trica."

Trica went and sat down. "How long y'all been here?"

"Not too long," Deb said. "You 'bout ready to come back to the big D?"

"Anytime. How Aunt Kitty doin'?"

"She's fine. Still 'round there eatin' all she can get."

Trica laughed. "That's Aunt Kitty for ya."

Mama said to Trica, "We got to have a talk when y'all finish playin' cards."

"Yes, ma'am."

Trica was crazy about Randy. Every time I looked at her, she was cuttin' her eyes at him. He never paid any attention to her though, not while anybody was around, but things were different when they were alone.

Gent went to the cabinet and took out a box of Kraft Deluxe macaroni and cheese.

She looked at me and said, "Hey, Head. You gonna throw this together for us?"

Before X could say anything, Deb jumped up and said, "I'll do it."

They played cards for hours. After they finished, Randy and Trica got missing for a while. We knew something was going on between them. He tried to hide it more than she did, but we knew better. They were so busy giving me a hard way to go that nobody paid any attention to them.

Charlie looked at me and shook his head. "Girl, you 'bout to pop," he said.

"She is mighty big, ain't she? For us to be havin' 'em at the same time."

"She might got her time mixed up. Do ya know when ya got pregnant?"

"Time a tell," I said.

"You ain't wrong about that. You might be havin' twins," Deb said.

"Girl, don't talk like that."

Mama said, "Well, that's whatcha wanted. I ain't never seen nobody that crazy in all my days. I was twenty-two before I got pregnant and didn't want none then."

"I didn't either. When the people told me that ma test was positive, I went back and asked Head what did it mean."

"I swear. Ya already got three youngerns and still don't know what it mean?"

"I do now."

Deb said, "That's a shame, ain't it?"

Gent said, "I got another good joint here. Y'all wanna smoke it now?"

"Might as well."

"Y'all better stop smokin' so much of that stuff and pregnant."

"It ain't gon' do nothin'," Gent said.

I agreed with her.

"All right. If them babies don't come out lookin' right, don't say that I didn't tell y'all."

THE FIRST CASE OF LUPUS

Mama kept fussing.

Trica came in and said, "I declare, ya up fussin' first thing this mornin'."

"I might as well hush. They ain't payin' me no attention anyway."

"They hardheaded, ain't they, Miss Nank?"

"Yeah, you can't tell 'em nothin'."

Gent had a bad habit of laughing at people. No matter what their problem may be, she made a joke of it. Mama always said that, if you laughed at somebody or teased them while you were pregnant, you could mark your baby.

They always talked about it happening back in the olden days.

We ate breakfast after everybody washed up, and we left around eight or nine. Mama was ready to get back home.

One thing she didn't do was stay away from home too long. No matter how good the hands were left with.

We got back, and Trica went back to live with Aunt Kitty. She still came to the house every day. It was like she was still there. She and Randy had some good times whenever they could sneak in a few minutes behind our backs.

A few weeks after we got back home, on December 30, I went into labor. I had a baby boy at four thirty-six that day. Mama called Gent and told her about it.

She said, "What! She left me, didn't she?"

"Yep. She gotta little big-head boy."

"Who do he favor?"

"Bobby Gene. He got her head and red for now."

"I swear I feel like cryin'."

"For what? Yo' time comin'."

"Did she raise much sand?"

"Child, no. I ain't never seen nobody have a baby that easy for it to be her first one."

"Well, that's good. My doctors told me that I ain't had no business gettin' pregnant with this lupus I got. He said that there could be some problems, but I ain't had none yet."

"Maybe it won't be too bad. Just pray and ask the Lord to help ya."

"I do."

"Well, I just called to tell ya the news."

"Okay. How much did it weigh?"

"Seven pounds, eleven ounces. I'll talk to ya later."

"Okay. Bye."

Nine days later, Mama got a collect call from Charlie.

He said, "Hey, I call to tell ya that Gent's in the hospital."

"She gettin' ready to have the baby?" she asked.

"Yeah. I was on the job. Yodi called me and said that she had to call the rescue squad to pick her up. She said that her water had broke and she had started hurtin'."

"How she doin'?"

"It don't look good. The doctor said that her blood pressure shot up and they think they gonna have to take the baby. He said that she ain't open up none for the baby to come out. I don't understand it. He said that the bottom of her stomach was as hard as a brick. He don't know what caused it hisself."

"My God! That's the first time I ever heard anything like that."

"He said that he would wait a little while longer and see if things change. He said that he didn't wanna wait too long 'cause it could kill her and the baby." Then he got a quiver in his voice like he was about to choke up.

"My Lord!"

"He said that one of them might not make it, but he'd try his best to save both of them. I told him, if he has to make a choice, to save Gent."

"Well, if ya need me to come down there, call me and let me know."

"Well, right now, there ain't too much nobody can do. But I'll keep in touch and let ya know what I find out."

"Okay. I'ma call Hannah and Tab and tell them."

"All right, bye."

Charlie went back to where Gent was. When he got next to her bed, she grabbed the shirt of his uniform and held on with all her might. The harder he tried to get loose, the harder she pulled. A nurse came in to check on her. She helped him calm her down, then

THE FIRST CASE OF LUPUS

he left. She was carrying on so bad that anyone looking at her could almost feel the pain.

Mama called Aunt Hannah and Aunt Tab. Both of them said they were praying for her. But Aunt Hannah's prayers were special. It was like she knew God personally.

Aunt Hannah told Mama, "Have faith and trust in the Lord. He'll help ya in a time of need. I believe in Him. Just ask Him to help ya, and things'll be all right. The doctor had his say, so now let me go talk to my doctor, which is Jesus."

Mama wouldn't let anybody use the phone until she heard that Gent was all right. Thirty minutes after she talked to Aunt Hannah, the phone rang again. She thought it might have been Charlie, but it was Aunt Hannah.

She told Mama, "Don't worry, Nank. She'll be all right, and the baby will too." Then she hung up.

Mama said okay and hung up, still worried though.

It wasn't but three or four minutes after she talked to Aunt Hannah when Charlie called.

He said, "She got a little girl."

Mama screamed, "Thank you, Jesus! How she doin'?"

"She's fine. They didn't have to cut her or nothin'. When the nurse went back in the room where she was, the baby was halfway out. The doctor had to rush in there and catch her. I would've called ya earlier, but I had to make sure that her and the baby was all right."

"And both of 'em doin' good?"

"Oh yeah. I was kinda worried for a minute. They said that, since she had the baby, her blood pressure should get back to normal. I thought that Yodi would have a fit when they said that the baby was born. She came up here to check on her."

"Well, I'm glad it's over with. Let me call and tell everybody."

"The baby gonna have to stay in here awhile because she's premature."

"That ain't too bad. The worst part is over. So I'll talk to ya later. Bye." She hung up the phone and started crying and hollering, "Thank You, Jesus, for liftin' this burden up off me!"

She and Aunt Kitty was so relieved that they took out a half pint of Canadian Club and drank it straight. I looked at them in surprise.

She said, "I just gotta calm ma nerves."

Neither of them were drinkers.

Both of them were crying.

Aunt Kitty said, "The Lord is a wonderful man, ain't He?"

"Oh yeah. He sho made a way for me today, and I thank Him."

"Hannah said that everything was gonna be all right."

"She know Him well, don't she?"

"Yes, sir."

"Lord, I feel so much better now. Maybe her troubles will all be over now."

"I know that yours is, ain't they?"

"Yes, they is. She better not try to have no mo'. As hard a time she had wit this one, I wouldn't."

"Me either."

After she had the baby and was put in her room, she slept all night and half of the next day. When she woke up, she called home. I answered the phone.

"Congratulation!" I said.

"Girl, I ain't never hurted that much in my life. I won't too far behind ya, was I?"

"No. Nine days. Pookie was born on the thirtieth, and yours was born on the ninth. Whatcha gonna name her?"

"Charlie wanna name her Regina Marie. That's probably what it'll be, but we gonna nickname her Stank."

"Stank? Dern, that sound worse than Pookie."

She laughed. "Where Mama?"

"Gone uptown. She should be back in a few minutes."

"I might come home to stay after the baby get old enough to travel."

"That'll be good. That way, the kids can grow up together."

"Yep. I'ma try to find me a house somewhere close to Mama. Let me go. They brought the baby in to stay with me for a little while. Tell Mama that I called."

"Okay."

THE FIRST CASE OF LUPUS

Then we hung up.

Mama came in right after I hung up the phone. I told her that Gent had called.

She said, "Is she gonna call back?"

"She didn't say."

We didn't hear from her anymore until after she was released from the hospital. She called to let us know that she was home. They kept Regina, but she was improving more each day. Gent hated to leave her, but she knew that she didn't have a choice.

When she called, Mama asked her, "Where you at?"

"Next door."

"You know you ain't got no business out in that cold and just had a baby. Girl, is you crazy?"

"I just wanted to call and letcha know that I was home, God."

"Well, good. Now get back in that house before ya have a setback."

"All right."

"And the next time ya wanna call, let Charlie do it for ya."

"Yes, ma'am."

"Okay. Bye-bye."

We didn't think she would call back anymore after what Mama told her, but she did the next day.

The first thing Mama said when she answered the phone was "What did I tell you, girl?"

She said, "I know whatcha told me, but this ain't no ordinary call."

"Why? What happened?"

After Gent had the baby, Trica went back to help her out when she came home from the hospital.

"Last night, some of Charlie's friends that he work with came over, and we got high. After they left, we went to bed. About one thirty or two o'clock, Charlie got up. I thought that he had to go to the bathroom, but he didn't. So I thought that maybe he was goin' to the kitchen to get him somethin' to eat, but he didn't go there either. I got up to see where he was goin'. When I got to the kitchen, I saw him standin' by Trica bed lookin' down at her. When I saw him reach for the cover she had on her, I said, 'Charlie, what in the hell is you doin'?' Then I turned on the light, and that's when Trica woke up. He said nothin' and that he was lookin' for a cigarette. I knew he was lyin' 'cause his cigarettes was on the table by the bed."

"What did he do then?"

"Nothin'. He went back to bed. It scared Trica so bad she couldn't hardly go back to sleep."

"I bet she was."

"Me and her sat up almost all night. She said that she wanted to go home 'cause she didn't want me to think that she had encouraged him to do that. I told her that I didn't."

"I think it'll be best if she come home. Ain't no tellin' what he had on his mind."

"No, there sho ain't."

"Another woman ain't got no business stayin' there anyway, unless it's his sister."

"That's right. Do ya wanna speak to her?"

"No. Just tell her to come on back home."

"All right, I'ma try to put her on the bus this mornin'. She don't wanna stay here another night, and I don't blame her."

"Me either. Let me know what time she get here so Sylvia Jean can pick her up."

"They'll tell ya that at the station."

"Okay."

"Okay, I'll see ya later."

They got Yodi to take them to the bus station. She wanted to know why Trica was leaving all of a sudden, but they didn't tell her. They told her that Trica's mother was sick and she wanted her to come home and help out with the kids.

I was at the bus station waiting for her when she arrived. She told me all about what had happened, but Gent and Charlie managed to work things out.

When Regina was a month and a half old, Gent moved back home with her. They stayed with us for a couple of weeks, and then she found a house not too far down the road from us. She talked to the man who owned it; and he told her that, if she wanted to stay in it, she could. She asked him how much the rent would be, and he said that she wouldn't have to pay anything because he didn't think the house was good enough to be lived in. He said that she'd have to fix it up herself, but she could stay in it as long as she wanted to.

The house was in a real mess, and it took a lot of hard work to get it fixed and clean. The whole yard was a trash dump. From the porch to the end of the yard, there was nothing but trash. The front porch had to be rebuilt. Grass had grown up to the windows. The backyard was just as bad as the front. The inside wasn't too bad, just nasty.

Joe found out that she was getting it, and he told her that he would help her out if she wanted him to. She knew that he was looking for something extra. She knew that she wasn't going to give it to him, but she said okay anyway.

I, Sterling, and Randy helped her get the yards straightened out. Mostly it was Sterling and I. Randy spent most of his time helping Joe with the porch.

In a week's time, we had it looking like a different house. Randy put in a hand pump. She tasted the water and told him to take it down because she didn't like the way it tasted.

He asked her, "Whatcha gon' do about gettin' water then?"

"Haul it from Mama's."

"That ain't gonna do nothin' but make a mess in the trunk of ya car. Then Charlie gonna pitch a bitch."

"No, he ain't. Shit, I gotta have water."

"Well, I reckon ya know." He went and took it down.

It was now starting to look like a home. We washed the windows and hung the curtains. We put strips of rugs on the floor. She couldn't afford a new one and arranged the little bit of furniture that had been given to her.

Saturday, she was ready to move in. Mama told her that she didn't think that she was going to let the baby go.

Gent said, "How come?"

Mama said, "Ya got any wood? Just because it ain't that cold that don't mean that, that baby don't need a fire on her."

"Randy cuttin' wood today. He said that he would bring me a load."

"Oh, what about food? Ya got any?"

"A little bit. Charlie get paid Monday. I should get mine in the mail Tuesday if he send it off Monday."

"Why don't cha wait till then to move in?"

"I can make it till then."

"And you can wait till then too." She got up to get a piece of wood to go in the heater. "That way, you can go on and do whatcha gotta do, and when ya move in, ya won't have to worry about it."

Gent just said, "All right," and played with the baby.

Mama tried to change her mind, but by the end of the day, she was all moved in. The house had four rooms. She didn't use the back bedroom. She said that it was too cold in it. When it was really cold, she'd stay at our house.

She tried to get one of her older kids to stay with her, but they didn't want to leave Mama, not even for a night.

Joe would come by every chance he got, but she told him to cut it out because people talked too much in Riverdale. They'd have it looking like Joe was staying with her and Charlie was taking care of both of them. He didn't want to stop, so he just cut it down to coming twice a week.

On the weekend of her birthday, March 26, she went to Georgia to spend it with Charlie. She left the Friday morning before her birthday.

Early the next morning, we got news that Joe had died. He'd had a heart attack. He was at home when it happened. The news shocked everybody. I knew that Gent would be hurt too.

When she got back the following Sunday night, I told her, "I know you gonna miss Joe."

"Why? Whatcha mean?"

"He died Saturday mornin'. He had a heart attack."

Her mouth dropped open, and she couldn't say anything for a while. "I know you lyin'!"

"No, I ain't either. Ask Mama if ya think I am."

She went in the room where Mama was. "Tell me it ain't true."

THE FIRST CASE OF LUPUS

"Well, it is. He was home when he died."

Gent leaned back on the wall and shook her head. "I seen him at the store Friday mornin' when I was on ma way to the bus station. I never thought that it would be ma last time seein' him."

"Ya never can tell where death is at. They said that he was on the phone when it happened."

"I know it liked to kill Dale and Beep Beep when they found out."

"Oh yeah, that was they buddy. It hurt all of us though."

"I still can't believe it. When he saw me at the store, he said, 'You tell Charlie that I'ma letcha go this time, but he better not look for ya to go no mo'.'"

"Yep, he's gone now."

"I got to get me somethin' to calm ma nerves now."

She left Mama's room and went back in the den. Randy got up, and they talked about it some more. For Gent, it was a hard pill to swallow. Joe had done a lot for her, and he let her know that she was always going to be number one in his life, even if she was married.

The next day, after ball practice, we went to the funeral home with his brother Ricky. All of his family was there. We went in and looked at him, and Gent started to cry. I waited until I got outside to cry.

When we got out to the car, she said, "Well, I ain't got no choice but believe it now. It's true. It's damn sho true."

"Yep, look like he just lyin' there sleepin'," I said, wiping tears from my eyes.

After we left the funeral home, she had Ricky take her to Deb's house. She got her a bag of weed and rolled three joints.

She said, "Hey, man, you don't mind if I light this up, do ya? I gotta settle ma nerves some kinda way."

"Go 'head. I don't mind. I know that you and Joe was old lovers, so I know how ya feel."

"Yeah, I'ma miss havin' him around."

"We all will."

When we left Deb's, Ricky went by the liquor store and got him a pint of Crown Royal. I guess that was his way of calming his nerves.

Gent took a couple of swallows of it too. No matter how much they drank or smoked, they didn't feel it. The hurt was there, and there was nothing that could take it away.

Gent wasn't able to go to the funeral. Her knees and ankles were stiff and swollen, which wasn't strange. She had trouble with them every month. The doctor told her that it came from the medicine she had been taking for lupus.

Next month, we started setting out tobacco. She didn't have any aches or pains the whole time we did it. We didn't think that she'd be able to work because it was cold in the mornings, our feet got wet while pulling plants, and sometimes it would be cold all day. But she never complained about any pain.

When the tobacco got up to the right size, we had to sucker it. That was a job breaking those unwanted blossoms out the top of each plant. Gent told Mama that she was going to help and that she could tend to the babies.

Mama said, "That's a lot of walkin'. Do ya think you can stand it out there in the sun doin' all that bendin'?"

"I had to bend to pull the plants."

"Yeah, but it won't as hot as it is now, and ya got to do a lot mo' walkin'."

"I'ma have a hat on. When I get too hot, I can sit down and rest."

"Child, it's up to you."

Two days later, we started. She did pretty good for a day and a half. On the second day, when we came home for dinner, she was coming up on the porch with her jacket and cap in her hand. She stepped up with the leg the doctor got the bone marrow from. We were already in the house, and we heard her on the porch hollering.

"Randy! Come here, Randy!" She was holding on to the pole.

Randy ran out and picked her up and brought her in the house. Mama was behind him.

She asked, "What happened?"

"Ma leg gave out on me. I couldn't move. Feel like it was stuck there."

THE FIRST CASE OF LUPUS

"I thought that it was cured. Ya think ya should go to the doctor and have him look at it?"

"No, it'll be all right. I thought it was well too."

"Maybe all that walkin' is what did it."

"It mighta."

"Well, I'll go back, and you can stay with the youngerns."

I said, "You ain't gotta go back. We ain't got nothin' to do but the little field. We'll get through with that early."

"Okay, I didn't wanna go anyway."

"I know it."

"Get ma money for me when ya go back," Gent said.

"It sho ain't take y'all long to get them three fields."

"Shine, we don't be playin'. We be gettin' down. Aunt Kitty is the only one out there creepin'."

"Leave my sister alone. She doin' the best she can."

We laughed.

We went back to work and were finished early that evening. When we got home and gave Gent her money, she had me take her to Deb's to get her a bag.

Mama said to her, "You ought to stop puttin' every penny you get in that shit. You coulda took that money and got that baby some Pampers or somethin'."

"She got Pampers. Her daddy gon' send me some money. I'll get 'em then. I'ma enjoy what I worked for."

"That's you. If he don't, don't look for me to get 'em."

"I won't."

She knew that Mama was just talking, but she was right.

The next week, Gent was waiting for the money. When she didn't get it in the mail, she called him to see what had happened. He told her that he was coming home that weekend and that he'd give her some then. Friday morning, she had to ask Mama to get Stank some Pampers.

Mama said, "What did I tell ya? The next time, you'll listen to me." Mama went on and got them.

Friday night, Charlie got home around ten. He told her that he was going to leave the car for her to have a way around. He said that she could pay the insurance and stuff when he sent the money. She was glad to hear that. That meant more money for her.

It wasn't long before he had to go back. Gent and I took him to the bus station. We took Stank with us to see him off. He played with her until the bus got there. As it drove up, he kissed her and Gent goodbye. Then he got on the bus and left.

He sent the money home to her like he said he would, but the bills weren't always paid. The insurance on the car was canceled a time or two because she hadn't paid it.

Then she'd go to Mama, and Mama would get the money to pay it for her. A lot of times, she wouldn't pay the light bill until it doubled. Mama would talk to her about it, but it didn't do any good. Each month from then on, she'd do the same thing.

It was now 1982. Gent and I were pregnant again. Charlie was out of the army and staying at home, and Stank and Pookie were going on three. Gent was due a month before me. She was due in August, and I was due in September.

We worked in tobacco that summer, and ray pregnancy went along well. In June, when we first started putting in the first crop, Gent was driving the tractor. She drove.

She drove for four days. When we went back on the fifth day, we walked to the field while we were waiting for the first drag.

She said, "Ma water broke last night."

"Why you didn't go to the hospital?"

"Because that's all that happened. I don't hurt or nothin'. Ma water just broke."

"You ain't said nothin' about it to Charlie?"

"No. I didn't see no blood or feel no pain, so I didn't say nothin' to nobody."

"You might have to go to the hospital for that."

"Yep, I always thought that, when ya water break, that meant ya was in labor."

"I did too."

"I'm peein' now." She held up her pants leg so I could see the water running down her leg. "I been flowin' like this all night almost. I pissed up the bed, and it's been runnin' down ma leg all mornin'."

THE FIRST CASE OF LUPUS

They came out the field with the drag, and we got on it and went to the barn. When the drag got to the barn, she got off and took her sheets and went back to the field.

I told Aunt Kitty what she had told me. When Sally, our other tractor driver, came to the barn, Aunt Kitty told her to tell Gent to come to the barn.

When she got there, Aunt Kitty said, "Whatcha tryin' to do? Kill yaself?"

"No."

"Don't cha think ya need to getcha self checked out if ya water broke?"

Everybody at the barn started getting on her for working in that condition.

"Yes, ma'am. When I go home for dinner, I'ma go."

Everybody said, "Ya better not wait till then."

Aunt Kitty said, "Ya better get somebody to take ya home now, or call Charlie and tell him to come and getcha."

"He workin'."

"I know, but can't cha call on the job and tell him thatcha need to go to the doctor or somewhere?"

"Yeah, Mama got Randy's car. She can take me."

"Ya still ain't hurtin'?"

"No. I ain't never had this problem before. With my first three kids, the only problem I had was that two of them was premature, and that won't by much."

"Maybe yo' sickness causin' it. Yo' body went through a lot and still goin' through it."

"That might be it." She went to the barn door. "'Kay, what time ya goin' to the store?"

"In a few minutes."

"I wantcha to take me home."

"What's wrong witcha?"

"I'm goin' to the hospital. Ma water broke, and I wanna see what the deal is."

"Well, we better go now then."

"No, you can finish this drag. It broke last night. I don't hurt or nothin'. I wanna see what caused it."

"Okay."

We finished it, and they left.

When we got home for dinner, Teresa was there with the kids.

Aunt Kitty said, "Nank and Gent still at the doctor?"

"She didn't go to the doctor. She went to the hospital. They gonna keep her. Nank said that they was gonna have to put her in labor."

"I figured they was gon' keep her. Did Nank say if she was gonna call back when we got home for dinner?"

"She said she'd call and let us know what happen."

A few minutes after we started eating, the phone rang. Teresa answered. It was Mama. She handed Aunt Kitty the phone.

"Hey," said Mama.

"Hey, how she doin'?"

"She had the baby. It was a little boy, but it didn't make it."

"My Lord. How Gent takin' it?"

"It hurt her, but she doin' all right. I'm gettin' ready to go home. I call Charlie, and he on his way up here."

"All right."

"I'll bring somethin' to make some sandwiches with and some sodas."

"We eatin' somethin'. I'll see ya when ya get here."

They hung up, and in a few minutes, Mama was pulling in the yard.

When she came in, I said, "What did Charlie say when ya told him about the baby?"

"He didn't say too much."

"Who did he favor?" asked Aunt Kitty.

"Stank. He looked just like Stank."

When Charlie walked in the room where Gent was, he looked at her in a strange way.

She said, "What's wrong with you?"

"What's wrong! What did ya tell yo' mama to tell me?"

"I know what I told her to tell you."

THE FIRST CASE OF LUPUS

"Then why did you ask what was wrong? This was what we wanted, a son, and he didn't make it. Maybe it just won't meant to be." He got quiet for a while. "Who got the body, Mrs. Page?"

"Yeah, he lived for about ten minutes after I had him."

"If he lived that long, he shoulda made it. They didn't try to save him. They coulda if they wanted to."

"You can't say that now. The Lord coulda took me just like he took the baby."

"I know that. But he lived for ten minutes. This just a sorry damn hospital. If I can help it, I don't ever wanna come here for nothin'."

"You gon' handle the burial arrangements?"

"When ya gonna do it?"

"Ya might as well go on and do it now. Ain't no use in waitin'. Go to the funeral home and pick out the little box. Ask for Dennis."

He came in and talked to them together. They had to have a place to bury the baby, and the man said that he could be buried at the foot of a relative's grave. Gent called Mama.

"Mama, Dennis said that we can bury the baby at the foot of somebody that's dead in the family. That way, we won't have to pay for a plot."

"Well, put him at the foot of Ma's grave. Somebody got to show 'em where it's at, and it sho ain't gonna be me."

"I'll call Deb and see if she'll go with them."

"All right, call me back and let me know what she said."

She called, and Deb said that she would go. They had the baby in a box the size of a shoebox. He was wrapped in a hospital blanket, and the hole they put him in wasn't very deep. They named him Luther Taylor Jr.

The next day, Gent got out of the hospital. The people on Charlie's job gave him a card to go to the florist to pick out a flower wreath of his choice for $20.

He had to work, so Gent and I did it. She named it little Charlie, after the baby.

She didn't go back to work for three weeks. Mama didn't want her to go then. She believed in keeping a person in bed for a month after having a baby. All she talked about was the baby and how my baby would be growing up by itself now. All of them said they'd have to spoil mine now. She looked forward to me having mine even though hers didn't make it.

Gent always said that she was going to go with me when I got ready to have my baby. On September 2 at four thirty in the morning, I started having labor pains. Ludy was on her way to work at Hardee's, so I called her and told her to give me a ride. She came by and picked up me and Mama, and we got Gent on the way out.

She didn't know what to think. When she got in the car, she said, "You sho pick some hellafied hours to go into labor."

I said, "I didn't put maself into labor. It was just time."

At twelve o'clock, I gave birth to a four-pound-and-six-ounce baby girl. Gent was in and out the whole time. She didn't leave until I had her. We made a bet. She wagered it would be a boy. She lost and never paid up.

For three years, things went pretty good for Gent and her family. Then came the year 1985. We like to lost her. She got pregnant with her sixth child. She went to the clinic and took a pregnancy test. They checked her medical records and found out about the trouble she had with her last two kids. She hoped, ever since she thought that she was pregnant, that she could get on the high-risk program. They put her down on the list to be certified.

The people in Florence at Memorial Hospital checked her records and got back in touch with the clinic. They wrote Gent a letter saying that she was accepted as a high-risk patient. They told her that she'd have to go to Florence Memorial Hospital for her checkups. She had to go once a week. Most of the time, she had to go on Thursdays. At first, they said that she would be going in a van, but it turned out that she had to get her own way there. When Randy didn't take her, I did.

We drove Randy's Grand Prix because Charlie's Cutlass couldn't make it. When Randy didn't want us to use his car, which was only once, she didn't go. She talked to Charlie about getting another car, and he did. He got an Electra 225. She didn't have to worry about getting there now.

THE FIRST CASE OF LUPUS

The first few times she went, they told her that her blood pressure was high. They gave her a prescription for some blood-pressure pills. She took them like she was supposed to, but they didn't seem to do any good. She kept taking them anyway.

In August, during her sixth month, she missed two appointments. She couldn't go because her feet were so swollen that she couldn't wear her shoes, not even her flip-flops.

When she did go back, they were talking about keeping her.

The doctor said, "You haven't been resting like I told you, have you, Jeanette?"

"Yeah, I been restin' some."

"Well, it's not enough. That's why your feet and ankles are so swollen. I'm thinking about keeping you for a while. Your blood pressure is still up too. But I'll let you go back home and stay another week and see how things turn out."

"Thank you, Jesus. I sho didn't wanna stay up here."

"Well, you better try to get some rest, or next week, you will have to stay."

She came out and told me that she was ready. On our way back to the car, she told me what the doctor said.

Then she said, "Girl, you know I'ma go home and get all the rest that I can 'cause I sho ain't ready to come up here and stay, not until ma time come to have it."

"How much rest ya plannin' on gettin' wit Stank there witcha?"

"Not too much, that's for sho. That little bit of time she be gone to school, I don't even miss her."

"Butcha enjoy that little bit of peace and quiet, don't cha?"

"You think I don't? I hope that they don't keep me when I come back next week, but if they do, I wantcha to send Stank to school for me."

"Okay, no problem."

When it was time for her next appointment, she didn't keep their car because she didn't have any money for gas. She went to Mama's to see if she could help out. But Mama didn't have any money either, so she had to miss another appointment.

Deb came by later on that day and said that she would have taken her if she had let her know earlier. It was too late to go then, but Gent asked her if she would take her for her next one. Deb said that she would.

So next Thursday, Deb was there early. She had Ludy with her. It took them a while to check her, and Deb was in and out trying to see what was taking them so long. It irritated Gent, and she wished that she had had somebody else to take her. She went and sat down for a little while. They had been there for two hours, and when the nurse came back to her desk, Deb asked her how much longer would she be back there. The nurse said that she didn't know and that the doctor was thinking about keeping her.

She didn't stick around to find out for sure if she was going to be admitted. She just told the nurse to tell her that she was gone and that she'd tell her husband that she was staying.

She turned to Ludy and said, "Let's ride."

Ludy said, "You ain't gonna wait and see what room they put her in if they keep her?"

"No. They can find that out when they come and see her."

"I thought the woman said that they might keep her."

"As high as her blood pressure is and as big as she swole, I know he ain't gon' send her home like that. And if they do, as long as it's takin' them somebody else, I'll be up here by then, and they can take her home."

Ludy got up and went with her because she didn't want to be left up there too.

When they got back, they came by my house and told me that they had kept her.

I asked them, "What room is she in?"

Deb said, "I don't know. They hadn't put her in a room when we left."

"Oh, they didn't say how long they was gonna keep her?"

"A couple of days. Just long enough to get her blood down and to get some of that fluid out of her."

"That's good. Ya told Mama yet?"

"No. I'm on my way back there now."

THE FIRST CASE OF LUPUS

"All right, I'll see ya later."

They told Mama. When Charlie got off work, they went to see her. She told Mama about how Deb was rushing and saying that she had to go and how she left before she knew that they were gonna keep her. Mama told her not to worry about it because she knew how her sister was.

The first two days went well. They got most of the fluid out of her, but they couldn't get her blood pressure down. It seemed to get higher. It was so high now that it made her feel dizzy.

On her third day, Charlie got off early to go see her, and Mama went with him. When they got there, the doctor told them that he was going to have to take the baby. He said that it was the only way he could get her blood pressure down. That worried Charlie because he had been through that before with Stank.

Mama and Charlie came back home to get her some more clothes and told us about Gent. When they got back to the hospital, they were all prepared to give her the shot to put her out, but they let them talk to her first.

They took her into the delivery room at twenty after six. Charlie paced and worried the whole time. Mama was sitting in a chair about to go to sleep.

Every time she dozed off, Charlie would say, "Ya reckon she doin' all right? They sho been in there a long time. Ain't nobody come out yet."

Mama would sit there with her eyes closed and say, "She all right. If anything woulda went wrong, they'da came out here and told us."

"Yeah, I didn't think it would take 'em this long."

"Oh yeah, they had to cut her."

He got quiet, and Mama dozed off. He left and took a walk down the hall. He looked at the clock, and it was now eight. He went back to the waiting room where Mama was and started pacing again.

He said, "Well, it's eight o'clock now. She done been in there almost two hours, and we ain't heard nothin' yet. I know they shoulda been took three or four babies by now."

"They gon' have you up here for high blood if ya don't sit down and stop worryin' about Gent. I told ya that she was gonna be all right."

When the doctor came in, he said that it was a little girl, and she weighed two pounds.

Charlie asked, "Is she gonna make it? That's a little small for her to make it, ain't it? And how's my wife?"

"She has a pretty good chance. Her heartbeat is strong, and everything is normal. I think she'll make it. And yes, your wife is doing very well."

"Can we see her?"

"Yes. They're putting her back in her room now."

They went to see her. She was still out of it.

Mama said, "She'll sleep the rest of the night."

Gent could hear them, but it sounded like they were far off.

The next day, Charlie went back. Mama and Aunt Kitty went with him. She was watching TV.

Mama said, "How ya doin'?"

"Pretty good. Glad it's over with."

"You ain't the only one. Ya seen the baby?"

"They brought her in this mornin'. I'm glad I won't have to go through this no mo'."

"What, he tied ya tubes?"

"And clipped 'em. He said that he was gonna stop me once and for all."

"Good. Ya didn't need no mo' anyway."

"Well, I ain't got that to worry about now."

Gent stayed in the hospital for two weeks. It took them that long to get her blood pressure down, and the lupus started getting worse. When she came home, she was taking high blood pressure pills and water pills. They had her on prednisone, but this time, the pills were bigger.

They told her to come back in four weeks for a checkup. She didn't go until her medicine ran out. She went back to see the baby every chance she got.

THE FIRST CASE OF LUPUS

When she did go back, she went to get a prescription for her prednisone. He told her that she didn't need one and that he didn't mean for her to keep taking them.

"That's why the water pills aren't working. It's the prednisone that has you swollen the way you are. Don't take any more of them. Take the water pills and the blood-pressure pills. You could have gone to your family doctor instead of coming all the way up here."

"Well, we came to see the baby, and I wanted to come and see about ma medicine."

"Well, just get that blood pressure back to normal, and you'll be in perfect health."

She left feeling a little better. But she knew that would always be a problem for her. The doctor said that, if she took too much of the prednisone, it would stiffen her joints. She and the baby, Thelma Novella, were doing fine; but even today, she still had stiffness in her joints. Lupus would always be a problem for her, but thank God she was living.

After weeks of not taking the prednisone, her body seemed to be shutting down. She had no energy to do anything. The only thing she wanted to do was lie around.

She wanted to hold the baby and spend time with her, but she couldn't. Charlie took her back to the doctor and told him how she was reacting to being off of the medicine. They had to put her back on it but had to gradually get her off of it, like taking a baby off of a bottle.

Things got better over time. They nicknamed the baby Bark. She came home and grew up to be a beautiful child.

The years passed. The kids were growing up. I was married to Bobby. Gent and Charlie were having marital problems, and the lupus only got worse. Gent was so sick that sex was the last thing on her mind. She could understand that Charlie was a man with needs, and she couldn't fulfill them anymore. She told him to just find him somebody else. He told her that he didn't want anybody else, but a man gon' be a man. He did just that but tried to do it on the down low. When she found out about it, she told him it was all right, but he needed to do it without her. So he moved back home with his parents. They had a good understanding about the situation, but Mama didn't.

Mama said he did her wrong and left her when she was sick. We didn't see it that way. She was sicker when he married her, but he was there for her. We knew that he loved her.

He always came around to check on his family. Gent lost the use of her legs. She couldn't walk. She had to wear briefs, and she had to go on dialysis because her kidneys quit. After that, things took a change for her and me. I took care of her like she was my baby, and in a way, she was. Whenever she needed changing, I was there. Mama didn't have the stomach to do it, so she'd call me. Even though I was married and out on my own, I was there whenever she called. They got her a power chair, and she was all over Riverdale with that thing. I had to get her off the side of the road a few times. She either had a flat tire or the battery was dead. She was sick, but it didn't keep her down. She was the life of the family. Her spirit kept us all laughing.

The first time Gent went into a coma and had to be rushed to the hospital, we didn't know what the doctor told her about keeping up her appetite, but he made sure she got something to smoke if she said that she hadn't eaten anything. Most of the time, she'd tell him that just to get something to smoke. We made sure she kept that. She'd get high and laugh about how she and Bobby Gene used to get Mama's car when he was 'bout drunk. Mama would tell him no, but Gent would get it anyway. She loved her Bobby Gene.

She took care of Uncle Vimp when he had to come and stay with Mama. He had dementia and was up and going with it. They had to go get him one day from somewhere in North Carolina. They found Mama's name on some mail he had in his car. Some kind of way, they got in touch with her and told her how to get to where he was. That's when she moved him in with her. Gent was doing pretty good during that time.

It wasn't long after he came that he turned for the worst and passed on.

Gent had to go to the doctor for a checkup, and they found out that she had ovarian cancer. They had to do a hysterectomy. She got ready to come home from the doctor's office. When they told her,

THE FIRST CASE OF LUPUS

she was crying. The word *cancer* scared her more than what she was already dealing with.

She had the surgery and came to Mama's. I had to take a long wooden Q-tip swab and stick in the place where they cut her and swab out the wound so the old blood could run out. I had to do it every day until the doctor said all of the blood was out. After she healed from that, that's when she started losing the use of her legs and she got the power chair.

Randy started calling her hot wheels. When she came through, you'd better be trying to get out the way. She ran over Mama one time and put a big gash on her leg.

Whenever she'd come to my house, she would be in the highway. We tell her not to be in the road.

She'd say, "They see me. They better not hit me," and wouldn't move.

When Gent started her kidney treatments, they put the catheter in her neck. It looked so painful. She complained all the time about it. One day, it started bleeding, and they had to rush her to the hospital in Florence. Her organs were shutting down, and they had to put her on a ventilator.

She stayed in the hospital on it for a week. They called all the family in the following week because the doctor was taking her off.

We were crying and praying. And again, God answered our prayers. She was breathing on her own, and her vital signs were improving.

They put her in a regular room. We were all waiting to see her.

When she woke up, she asked, "Where is Bark baby?"

I said, "What baby? Bark ain't got no baby."

"Is Aunt Hannah dead?"

"No. You sho been doin' a lot of dreamin'," said Randy.

"Boy, I done seen all kind of stuff. But Bark had a baby boy."

She came home, and as time passed, she didn't seem to get any better. But she wasn't getting any worse either.

She couldn't walk or do too much for herself, but she was hanging in there, smoking as much weed as she could. That seemed to help her more than the medicine. She could no longer roll her own joints, so we had to do it for her.

After our kids got up and were almost grown, they all started smoking too. By the time they started, they had stopped smoking joints and started smoking blunts, taking the tobacco out of the cigar and refilling it with weed.

I went over to Mama's one day to see Gent; and she, Sterling, Tula, and Granny was smoking a blunt. When I walked in, Gent passed it to me. I took a hit and passed it back to her.

"Don't pass it to me. That's Granny's."

"Who?" I said. I didn't even know that she smoked.

Granny was so shocked the only thing she did was take it like nothing new was happening.

Gent laughed and said, "Well, if she didn't know, she do now. Hell, pass the blunt."

She was fifteen. I didn't say anything. I started when I was twelve.

Time passed, and so did a lot of people. The year was 2000. Granny had a little boy the day after New Year's, my first grandchild.

Two months after he was born, Mama had a stroke at the brain. Aunt Essie was home at the time, and she called me at three o'clock in the morning. She told me to come and check Mama's blood pressure because she wasn't acting right. When I got there, they were in Mama's room on the bed. She could hardly get her words straight, and it sounded like her tongue was heavy.

"This don't look good," I said while putting the blood pressure cuff on her arm.

Her reading was 224/130.

I didn't bother calling the EMT. We got her in my car with the help of the good Lord, and I took her to the hospital. That was one heavy little woman. She couldn't stand or help us out no way whatsoever.

They kept her in the hospital for three weeks. She was out of it for a while. I went by there one day after work, and I heard her screaming. I ran to the door, and she was on the bed holding on to the rails screaming.

THE FIRST CASE OF LUPUS

"I'm fallin! I'm failin'!"

I ran to her and grabbed her around the shoulders. "No, you ain't. I gotcha," I said.

"Lord, ma head is just spinnin'! I'm failin'!"

"I gotcha. Just calm down. When ya head start spinnin', just close your eyes and lie back. Don't look up. Look down witcha eyes closed."

The nurses came in and asked me to leave out so they could check her. By the time I left out, there were a few more people in the hall waiting to see how she was doing.

They called the doctor in, and he ordered some tests to be done on her. The next day, they transferred her to Duke University Hospital in Durham, North Carolina. I took time off from work to go with her. I was there for two weeks. I told the nurse to just show me where everything was and I'd take care of her. They tried to give me a job there, but I told them that I had a sick sister and a sick mama to take care of.

After Mama had the stroke, Gent seemed to get a little worse. She was back and forth in the emergency room.

A month passed, and the spinning in Mama's head got a little better.

When the doctor made his rounds with his interns, Mama said, "I done been in here a month, and y'all ain't did nothin' for me. Every day, it's the same thing. I want you to send me home."

"I can't keep you here if you don't want to stay, but I can't send you home."

"Whatcha mean?" she asked him.

"I'll have to send you to a rehabilitation center."

"Where one of them at? Is there one in Dillon?"

"No, ma'am. The closest one is in Florence."

"That's close enough," she said.

While they were transporting her to Florence, I went home to get some rest. Later that day, Gent had to be admitted into the hospital right down the street from where she was.

Mama had a catheter in, and she had a tube feeder. After she got to Health South, it was like she got a lift on life. On the second day, they called my brother and told him that Mama was refusing treatment and said that she was going home. He told them that he would be up there in the morning because we had just left from seeing her and Gent.

The next day, we went. When we got there, Mama was sitting on the foot of her bed fussing. My brother and I looked at each other and shook our heads. We couldn't believe that she was up like that with a catheter and a feeding tube hooked up to her. She was so mad she looked at us like she could run through us.

We didn't tell her about Gent being in the hospital. She was in ICU and not doing too good. He told the people to get Mama's release papers ready and that we'd be back. We told them we were going to check on Gent but not to tell Mama because we didn't want to upset her.

We were in the waiting room waiting to go in and see Gent, and a nurse came in.

"Is there anyone here with the Casey family?" she asked.

"Yes, we are," I said.

"You have a phone call. You can pick up and mash 9."

I picked up the phone. "Hello?"

It was Mama. "How ma gal doin'?"

I couldn't believe it. "How you know she was in here?"

"You can't keep nothin' from me. How she doin'?"

"She doin' all right."

"They ain't said nothin' about her comin' home?"

"No, ma'am, not yet." Looking over at the others, I said, "This Mama."

"How she callin' checkin' on Gent and in the hospital herself? What we gon' do wit her?" asked Na.

"Well, come on. I'm ready to go," she said.

They got EMTs to take her home because she had so much hooked up to her. We were worried about how we were going to do this. I had to work. Our cousin who was a nurse came and did it the first time she got home. After that, Mama started peeing on her own. She still had to be fed by the tube, but after I took her to the doctor a week later, she got off of that too.

THE FIRST CASE OF LUPUS

Na said, "Look like all she had to do was come home, and she got better, like this house is her remedy."

Gent came home a week later. There was nobody at home with them now but Bark. The rest of them were out on their own. Between Gent and Mama, I was about to wear myself out.

I got off work every day and went to check on them. One morning, I had to give Mama a bath and was at the sink filling a pan with water to wash her and passed out. I fell flat on my back. I could hear what everybody was saying, but I was out.

Mama yelled, "What in the world was that?"

Stank ran in the house. "Aunt Silver Jean! What happened?"

She said that I had my hands behind my head like I was doing sit-ups. She, Tula, and Gent were on the porch smoking when I came up. I hadn't smoked in seven years, so I took a pull that morning before I went in the house.

Stank said, "We got to start helpin' you. Yo' body is tired."

Tula said, "I know she ain't smokin' no mo' weed wit me. She know she ain't been smokin'."

I went home and lay down. By the end of the day, I felt like I had been hit by a truck. I was so sore.

Years passed, and Gent's health went down. It was 2006 and the day before Thanksgiving. Gent had to be rushed to the hospital. Her sugar had dropped down to 11. The doctor said he didn't see how she was making it. They kept her in the hospital for a few days. We had to keep a record of it and her blood pressure.

Gent slept on sofa in the living room. She didn't get out too much in her chair anymore. She still smoked her weed though. She couldn't hold the blunt, so one of her girls did it for her.

We were talking one day, and she said, "You know, I seen a lot of people leave this ole world. Some of them thought I'd go first, but God didn't see it that way."

"You right. He the only one that know the time we gon' go."

"Just think about it. Joe, Bobby Gene, Aunt Kitty, my daddy, and so many mo'."

"And still might see some mo' go before you."

"You right," she said.

After Bobby got killed, it seemed like anything bad that could happen to me happened in February. Gent took a turn for the worse. It was February 8. They put her back in the hospital in Florence. When I went to see her, they were asking me all kinds of questions about who was her caregiver. They wanted to say she was being abused and said we weren't feeding her. I had to explain to her how that sickness did her. I told her that I was her caregiver and abuse was out of the question. This was the third time she had to be put on life support. I was her contact person, and when they called me to tell me that she was on it, my whole day was messed up. People at work kept asking me if I was all right. She was on it for a week.

When they took her off, she could breathe on her own, but she was still unresponsive. After a couple of weeks, she started talking.

The nurse called me on my job and said, "I have some good news for you," which was a relief.

When they told me that it was the hospital on the phone, my heart dropped.

"Oh, yeah."

"Yes, ma'am. Your sister asked for you."

"Thank God. Tell her I'll see her tonight."

"All right, I sure will."

I didn't get a chance to go that night. I had to do something after work. But the next day, that was the plan.

I called Deb to see if she'd be able to go with me when I got off. She said that she'd already be there. So I asked her husband, Howard, to go with me; and he said that he would.

My coworkers were teasing me all day, saying that was the happiest I'd looked all week and that they knew I was ready to get off and go see her. They let me leave an hour earlier.

When I pulled in the yard to pick up Howard to go to the hospital, he came to the door and held up a finger and said, "Wait a minute."

He came out to the car with his head down.

"That was Deb on the phone. Ain't no need in goin'. She gone. Deb said she just passed."

THE FIRST CASE OF LUPUS

My heart dropped. I just put the car in reverse and left. I had remarried, and he called my husband to tell him about Gent and that he had told me and to look out for me. When I got home, I walked into the living room, fell on the sofa, and let it out.

The next week seemed so long—making funeral arrangements and getting things together. Charlie was right there for his kids. He was still good in my point of view.

She had a big funeral.

I kept telling myself, "She ain't suffering no more."

That's how I made it.

CPSIA information can be obtained
at www.ICGtesting.com
Printed in the USA
LVHW100055050623
748714LV00031B/133

9 781636 929187